THERE IS A WAY

Sharon Bull

© Sharon Bull 2016

All rights reserved.

Sharon Bull has asserted her right under the Copyright, Designs and patents act 1988 to be identified as the author of this book.

No part of this publication may be reproduced, distributed, or transmitted in any form or by any means, without the prior written permission of the author, except in the case of brief quotations embodied in critical reviews and certain other non-commercial uses permitted by copyright law. For permission requests, contact the author.

ISBN-13: 978-1523855193

ISBN-10: 1523855193

Cover design © Socciones

Introduction page photograph © Steve Hill Photography

Design & formatting by Socciones Editoria Digitale

www.kindle-publishing-service.co.uk

MY GRATITUDE AND THANKS

This book would never have been written without the help of many people, so my gratitude and thanks goes out to all my family and friends living and past, who I love, treasure, and have had the pleasure to share my life with. Special thanks go out to my Mum, who without a shadow of a doubt has been my Guardian Angel, particularly during my darkest hours. My dear departed Father, who has always been my strength from being a little girl, which made it all the more difficult when he parted from this world. My younger brother Paul, his wife Joanne and my beautiful nephew Jude, cousins Sandy and Marg, my Dad's sisters Aunty Anne and Aunty Betty and my two dearest friends Marie and Margaret. I have met many inspirational people along the way, some who in turn have become great friends too, but I would also like to thank Alan Dolman, the first person to believe I could make something of myself, Squeeze, for encouraging me to make it happen and Paul Davies, my mentor for finally connecting all the dots. I would also like to show my appreciation to Deana Sampson, Jenni Fellows, Tracey Webster, Teresa Yates and Jeffery Caunt, who have all supported my work from the start. May I also take this opportunity to say thank you to everyone who has given me both the encouragement and strength to continue along this path.

'In loving memory of Kevin Anthony Bull'

Sharon Bull
www.acompassionatevoice.co.uk

INTRODUCTION
THIS IS THE STORY ABOUT ME

*'This is the story about me.
But what you might see and recognise within me,
Is perhaps a part of you too?'*

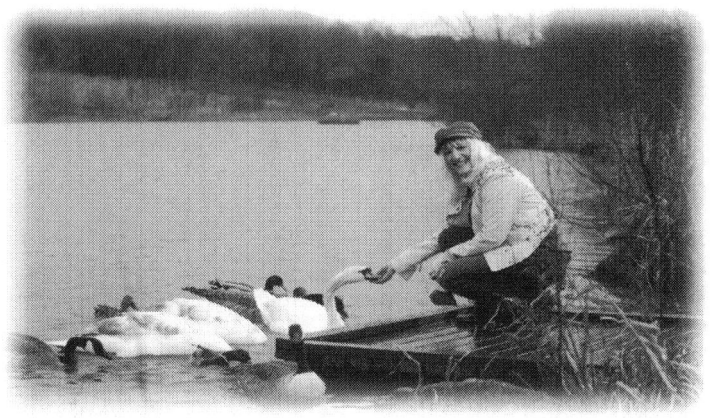

"In 2010 I woke up!"

It was an extremely difficult time for me because I lost almost everything, including my life. But it's in adverse times we grow and learn, even though we don't see it at the time.

In a book called 'How to be Compassionate' by the Dalai Lama he speaks about his own life. He quotes…

'In my own life, the most difficult periods have been the times when I have gained the most knowledge and experience.'

And I say I lost almost everything, because what remained after being stripped of all the superficial garbage that I perceived for thirty years to be the key to all happiness was me – my true authentic self.

I lost my job as a top sales executive with a British brand leader, my company car, wardrobe of designer clothes and shoes, credit cards, my home and consequently my self-respect, because I placed all this material stuff above everything else. How I thought I needed to look and how I thought I needed to be in society had somehow become the focus of my life. Sadly, this self-centred approach of my this, my that, my body, my car and my promotion affects so many of us, galvanised by years of cleverly constructed marketing, engineered by banks and large corporate businesses to make huge profits.

What baffles me the most about this time is how I couldn't see that my constant bouts of severe depression, anxiety, stress, low self-esteem and debt - a consequence of my spending addiction, were all painting a completely different picture, and it wasn't happiness!

Up until 2010, my mind was completely occupied by a self-cherishing attitude, a mentality that seems to be encouraged across western civilizations. We are constantly striving to be better than the next person by improving our status, climbing the ladder and accumulating material possessions, but at what cost? It is no surprise there is a rise in mental illness, when we are forever being persuaded by advertisers selling their latest products never to be satisfied with who we are and what we have. A sickness which has no boundaries, or prejudice as it weaves its way into schools, workplaces and all walks of life, including the rich and famous, young and old, male and female, poor and disadvantaged. The growth in mental health issues is frightening, which is why we need to ask ourselves why?

Just like every other living being sharing this planet, we enter this world with absolutely nothing and no matter how much wealth we may accumulate during our tiny spell here, it is worth remembering we still leave in the same way we arrived – with absolutely nothing.

I look back on my sixteen years in a sales career and realise I was never actually cut out to be the aggressive hard sell negotiator, but yet I had strived for such a long time to be in this type of post. I perceived it to be a glamorous role, one with a multitude of perks and high salary, however, what I hadn't considered was the long days, hours stuck in motorway traffic, or the numerous soakings caught in downpours as I trudged the streets weighed down with sample goods.

My situation became almost unbearable because whilst creditors called me around the clock for missed payments I was trying to keep up appearances in my working role. Rather than face the music, I buried my head in the sand wallowing in self-pity.

I do believe we are eventually sent warning calls to divert us from a path which is destroying our true spirit, it may be illness, redundancy, loss, or even a break up in a relationship and although this may seem totally unfair, a complete travesty, or injustice at the time, it can so often be our saving grace. I look back over the years to consider the countless obstructions, hurdles, difficulties, drawbacks and hindrances thrown across my path and wonder why my brain just didn't register the messages being sent.

My love of animals has been with me since being a little girl, but yet I never really considered that I could possibly help to make a difference for them. Perhaps being heavily influenced by a possession led mentality didn't help either, maybe I didn't feel they ranked high enough in my list of priorities. I now ask myself why, when saving the life of a flea battling to survive in the bird bath, is as equally important to me as caring for my thirteen-year-old cat Maddie.

I owe my life to wildlife and nature, because it was wildlife and nature that reopened my heart and reminded me who I truly was - a little girl who wouldn't shoo a pigeon, who spent most Sunday afternoons picnicking in the countryside, who grew up and even during her façade still wouldn't tread on a spider.

We live in a society fixated by status, competition and consumerism, yet it's through this type of thinking we can so easily become attached to a particular person, situation or object, believing this will open the door to a more fulfilling and happier life. The bigger house, the faster car, the next job promotion, or relationship – whatever external entity we perceive to be the conveyor of instantaneous happiness is merely a distraction, unless we are at peace with ourselves.

Competition isn't always a bad thing, however, when it becomes an obsession driven solely by greed and power it encourages a selfishness that has little, or no respect for others. Corruption, bullying and bestowing fear, pain or distress on any living being to achieve stature and material gain is certainly not the antidote to anyone's wellbeing and happiness, but neither is anger towards the perpetrators of ill deeds or people whose values seem different to ours. Judgement of others doesn't help, because there isn't one person, country or nation that can point the finger at another, without three fingers pointing back.

A few years ago, a wonderful lady called Alice Hertz Sommer was brought to my attention by a dear friend. Alice was a Prague born Jewish pianist, a music teacher who survived Theresienstadt concentration camp because of her musical talent. Saved from death, she continued her life's journey until February 23rd 2014 when she passed away at the age of 110, the oldest Holocaust survivor. Alice had an optimism for life, a generosity that knew no bounds, but her forgiveness and compassion was immeasurable, which was captured perfectly in all of her interviews.

> *'Hatred eats the soul of the hater not the hated.'* Alice Herz-Sommer

'Life is Beautiful' – a poem I wrote in 2012 was inspired by Alice's ethos in life and became the catalyst for many more of my future poems.

For thirty years, the genuine Sharon Bull played second fiddle to all the mad distractions I associated with being happy and it wasn't until I reached my lowest point I found what I believe to be my purpose. I had no idea how I was going to turn things around, however, a few years on and my work as an inspirational speaker, author and poet is encouraging others to overcome their own personal hurdles, helping to raise awareness about the importance of nature and wildlife for our well-being and enlightening people about the countless animal welfare issues across all corners of the world. Most importantly though, it has enriched my life in ways I could never have imagined.

There is a way, but we have to be the change we wish to see in the world first, then others will be inspired to follow and the only way we can do this is from the heart. We are all connected to nature and wildlife, equally though, we are all connected to each other, therefore unity, compassion and kindness is the only way we will ever see positive changes in the world we live in. If I can make these changes, anyone can, so although this book is about me, what you might see and recognise within me, is perhaps a part of you too!

After numerous requests for some of my poetry to be published, I have dedicated chapter 17 'A Compassionate Voice' to some of my more poignant verse.

CONTENTS

CHAPTER 1 - ONCE UPON A TIME 1
CHAPTER 2 - NO MAN WILL MARRY YOU! 8
CHAPTER 3 - THE NEXT THIRTY YEARS 14
CHAPTER 4 - THE FIRST SIGN 22
CHAPTER 5 - 150 MILES AWAY 29
CHAPTER 6 - BARKING MAD 40
CHAPTER 7 - THE BUTTERFLY SYMBOL 48
CHAPTER 8 - TRYING TO BUY HAPPINESS! 53
CHAPTER 9 - THE LAST FEW HOURS 63
CHAPTER 10 - SINGLE BED 74
CHAPTER 11 - EXCHANGE OF APPLES 83
CHAPTER 12 - TURNING POINT 94
CHAPTER 13 - NATURE HEALS 107
CHAPTER 14 - A NEW BREED OF POLITICIAN 121
CHAPTER 15 - THERE IS A WAY 127
CHAPTER 16 - ALWAYS CHOOSE LOVE 137
CHAPTER 17 - A COMPASSIONATE VOICE 147

CHAPTER 1
ONCE UPON A TIME

'She would tippy toe in Mummy's heels across the kitchen floor,
Red lipstick smudged across her lips
Pinched from her mummy's drawer.'

When I look back, I don't think I liked myself very much as a child. I seem to remember feeling clumsy, awkward and plain looking most of the time. Looking up to cousins, envious of school friends, especially the girls with long flowing, golden coloured hair. Mum, like most Mothers around the time of my childhood, kept my hair extremely short in her combat to keep the head lice away and as a little girl, I yearned to have my hair in a ponytail or plaits.

I don't recall too many early childhood memories, just a few snap shots flicker around in my mind and the recollections I do have almost feel like long forgotten pictures in a dusty old photo album. A compilation of fading images giving away barely any detail from the past, some may hold a few more clues and reminders, whilst others echo very little.

Playing a wonderful make believe game with Mum's personal belongings is perhaps one of my earliest memories. I was six years old when my infatuation with Marilyn Monroe started. I didn't dream about being a princess like most little girls, I just wanted to be like Norma Jean - a beautiful lady, who had transformed herself into a Hollywood movie star with stylishly curled blonde hair, a curvaceous body and an open ended wardrobe of desirable clothes. Tippy toeing around the family home in Mummy's high heels, I would mimic her red carpet walk, wearing bright lipstick smudged across my lips that was pinched from Mum's dressing table drawer. To me, an impressionable child, Marilyn was the epitome of beauty and elegance, who appeared to have everything her heart desired and yet, I began watching her movies four years after her death at 36. Was Marilyn happy? I doubt she was, even though her well documented glamorous lifestyle would seem to portray her as having it all.

Unbeknown to their two little ones, life had drawn my parents a raw deal during our infancy and by the mid-sixties we had moved home on more than one occasion. Being a small child, I probably didn't have any real concept of how tough the times were for Mum and Dad, and my brother being two years younger was probably even more oblivious to their plight. Now though, I question just how much I had taken on board as a little girl, wondering if this is possibly the reason why some of my earlier memories seem so difficult to recall. Please don't get me wrong, my brother and I were dearly loved and although our parents could rarely afford the best toys on the shelf, they always tried to make sure we never went without.

I attended a Catholic school during my primary years, where I was inspired regularly by Nuns, resulting in a fascination towards a vocation within the Church. Being only nine at the time, I have never been certain what the intrigue was, perhaps it was the attire they wore, or a curiosity about the convent and the life style they lived. Maybe I was influenced by our family babysitter Bridget, a wonderful young woman, who at that time was a novice nun preparing for her ordainment. One thing I am sure about though, the aspiration to be part of something holy had nothing to do with the Church, or the priests serving the parish at that time, as I found them both extremely intimidating.

For many years I have amusingly relayed my 'Sound of

Music' story at parties, jokingly declaring that the thought of wandering around quietly in a convent, adorned only in a habit and veil, without make-up, perfume and high heels was just too hideous to even consider. *'How do you solve a problem like Maria'*, would probably still be my anthem tune today. Should I reconsider my decision to join a holy sisterhood though, meditation, flat walking shoes and chilled down days without make up, or fuss isn't so out of character anymore.

If I am to be perfectly honest about the Church's impact on my childhood, then I would have to say I was never encouraged by the Sunday sermons, in fact most of the time I was either clock watching, or teasing my younger brother Paul. It was through this boredom and a natural inquisitiveness I began to notice a divide between the wealthy and working class of the parish. *'The fancy hats brigade'* I would secretly call them as a juvenile and it certainly left me with a bitter taste towards the church for quite a number of years. I would watch the upper class of the congregation trip over each other's feet, fighting for the first few pews at the front of the church, the husband dangling his flash BMW, or Mercedes car keys for everyone to see, as he walked down the aisle parading his wife in her big floppy hat. Walking behind them would be their perfect children, girls in bonnets and lacy gloves, the boys suited and booted, without a hair out of place.

As the Mass finally came to an end and the organ played out its final few notes, the parish priest always walked slowly down the church aisle, making his way towards the enormous porch entrance in order to greet his parishioners. Jumping out of their front row pews to follow at his heels, the fancy hats brigade shadowed him closely, so amusingly by the time Dad, Mum, Paul and myself reached the church's huge wooden doors, we would barely be able see the top of the holy Father's head, let alone receive his handshake.

Even at such a tender age, I reckoned spending an hour in a holy place once a week didn't constitute goodness in a person and neither did deep pockets entitle someone with an automatic first class ticket to heaven. Looking back, I think even as a small child I had almost figured it out, and I do recall grabbing hold of Dad's hand one Sunday morning as we stepped outside the church, to quiz him about religion. My little mind hadn't yet quite grasped humanities cravings for stature, importance and supremacy, so I was totally bemused by some of the parish's behaviour. Besides, the only convincing way I could see of obtaining a key to heaven's door was by always conveying love and kindness to others, and as Mum and Dad constantly lavished Paul and me with heaps of the stuff, in my eyes they certainly qualified as exceptionally good people. For me, I didn't think Jesus could be swayed, or influenced by the vast amount of money in someone's bank account, or I doubt he cared what brand of car a family drove to church in each Sunday morning either - if that was the case our ten-year-old Ford Cortina would never have made the grade.

I left a catholic education behind to further develop my chosen career path, a profession which had now deviated from nun to nurse and because of this I was accepted into a secondary school dedicated to this caring occupation. Attending a non-Catholic school made it so easy to turn my back on a religion I thought was steeped in bias and yet Christmas, Easter and even the odd sunny Sunday morning, I would proudly join my devoted Dad in his usual seat at the back of the Church.

Without a shadow of a doubt, school education plays a huge role in the moulding of our future adulthood. From a babe in arms, we are shaped into characters conditioned by parents, families and teachers, but is this who we truly are, or are we sometimes withholding our deepest desires and talents through a fear of not fitting into society? There is no one to blame and how often is it stated to people daring to question aged traditions, *'this is how it has always been!'* Generation after generation we pass down beliefs and teachings to children, some of which perhaps no longer serve the world, or the twenty first century we live in today.

From an early age we are so easily swayed, influenced and transformed to fit into our society, one which seems increasingly driven by consumerism and yet throughout our education we are not always made fully aware of what lies ahead, beyond the confines of the school classroom and playground. I can only go by my own experiences as a student and although I wasn't the most attentive pupil in my class, neither was I the least intelligent. Mathematics, English Literacy, Science, History and Geography understandably need to be part of the curriculum, however, within the academic timetable there has to be much more emphasis placed on the importance of our connection with each other.

If there are to be any positive changes in this world, young minds must also learn about difference, whether it is the colour of someone's skin, a disability, religious belief, or even an extraordinary talent. We need to understand at an early age that contrast shapes the planet we all share and no life is any less, or any more important than another. Lessons should include mindfulness, meditation, how to handle finance, health in body and mind, all key ingredients to our well-being and each of paramount importance for a stable, more fulfilling, happier life. Most significant of all, schools must encourage compassion and kindness, not only towards other living beings, but with regard to ourselves too.

Not long into my secondary education, I became the victim of a fifth form bully, who seemed to derive great pleasure from making younger students cry. My name was finally added to her score sheet when she punched me in the face at the school tuck shop. It wasn't so much the stinging on my cheeks from her fist why the tears fell, more the embarrassment of it being witnessed by her crowd of adolescent admirers, as they coaxed and encouraged her to deal the blow. Ashamedly, a few years later the tables were turned and I became one of the school bullies, whilst trying to portray a couldn't care less attitude towards three years of mediocre exam results, appertained through a lack of ambition for my future life ahead. Teacher intervention to deter the bully was either detention or a ruler to the hand, and for the bullied it was a simple suggestion to toughen up.

My sole purpose for attending this particular school had been to stay on into the sixth form and receive nurse training, however, this was soon quashed when I realised I couldn't stand the sight of blood and my priorities turned to boys. The school I attended was an all-girls establishment, but this didn't hinder our chances with the opposite sex, as there was never a shortage of admirers outside the gates from the two neighbouring schools.

After months practising with a settee cushion, my first real kiss was experienced at a party organised by myself and a school friend to celebrate our fourteenth birthdays. A local, older boy had caught my attention during the get-together and somehow the encounter had taken place underneath a piano in the room we had hired. For a number of weeks after the event I was constantly teased by school chums, but it didn't matter, I secretly enjoyed the attention and so from then on I let the educational system slip through my fingers, as my dreams shifted from finding the perfect vocation to finding the perfect man.

At fifteen I hit the bottle, not the whiskey bottle, the peroxide bottle and Mum's face was a picture when she first saw the results. She had always made it perfectly clear that until I left school bleaching my hair was against the rules, but rules were meant to be broken, and besides I couldn't wait that long. So, with some money put aside from my weekend waitressing job, I purchased the inexpensive do it yourself kit and the result was a disaster - a head full of bright canary yellow hair. Mum was beside herself when she returned home later that evening from a night out with Dad, but the damage was done and the only thing she could do was improve the situation. Fortunately, my cousin was a professional hairdresser with her own salon, so Mum booked me an appointment having no doubts Sandy would be able to restore my hair to a more natural blonde colour. This was what I had hoped for, my new grown-up look was here to stay, albeit toned down a little.

I was sixteen when I walked through the school gates for the last time and a few days later I sampled full-time employment, working as a shop assistant in a local convenience store. It didn't pay much, the owner spent most of his time either in the pub, or chatting up his younger female staff, including me, but it was my first taste of independence. It was also a testing time for me, because suddenly I didn't seem to know who I was anymore, or what I wanted from life.

CHAPTER 2
NO MAN WILL MARRY YOU!

'People look at me and see confident
They see relaxed and self-assured,
But behind this glint, behind this smile
I can tell you it's been a fraud!'

My job at the convenience store didn't last too long, because after being blatantly asked by the boss in my first meeting with him if I was on the pill, I knew I had to get out. The business collapsed a short while after I handed in my notice, which wasn't much of a surprise, as not long after my recruitment I realised that theft and corruption by some members of the staff was rife. The unopened red letters were already stacked high on the owner's desk before I left and seeing as he spent most of his working days getting inebriated in the pub, the odds of having a long and happy employment at the shop was hardly likely.

Packing drinking glasses into fancy packaging could sometimes be extremely tedious, but factory work paid out higher wages, I made some good friends, including my best friend Marie, and we still reminisce about the great times we had today. My weekly salary honoured my lifestyle more, just like most seventeen-year-old girls, nights out with work mates, new clothes and make up all became relatively normal expenses.

My ties with finding the perfect partner and marriage were severed when I fell upon new adventures through a love of live music, which was strengthened when watching a support band for Eddie and the Hot Rods in the late seventies called 'Squeeze.' From the moment they walked onto the stage that evening I was completely blown away, so for the next few years most of my leisure time was spent travelling the length and breadth of the country to see their gigs. The excitement of the shows, visiting new places and hanging out with professional musicians far exceeded pursuing husband material amongst local, spotty boys and besides, settling down with 2.5 children suddenly didn't seem so appealing anymore.

But it was in-between the concerts and back stage passes when the problems began to emerge and gain momentum. Dissatisfactions of who I was seemed to intensify, until without any warning a severe bout of mental illness descended over me, playing havoc with all my emotions and making me feel inadequate and worthless.

At first family and friends thought I was suffering from a spell of teenage blues, but when my parents returned home from a night out to find me cowering like a frightened child in the corner of the living room, they realised there had to be something much more sinister going on. The depression seemed to come from nowhere and yet its side effects certainly made their presence felt with panic attacks, heart palpitations, breathlessness and severe headaches. These were just a few of the symptoms that seemed to linger for months and months. Loved ones were often taken by surprise when in a moment's notice claustrophobia would induce me into running out of shops, cafes, and pubs, or irrational fear would prompt me into pressing the bell to disembark from a bus two or three stops before my destination.

Confused, frazzled, utter chaos, the only descriptions I can give about my mind at the time and the one explanation I have for its delicate state was a complete frustration with life. Mum made me an appointment with the family doctor, but after a few consultations I was still showing no signs of improvement in my poor mental state, so the GP referred me to a psychiatrist.

I believe this is when I formulated and embedded deeply into my thinking some extremely false perceptions about myself, which not only caused low self-esteem, but also misguided my decision making and helped to draft out the next thirty years of my life.

"No man will marry you looking like that; men don't marry women like you!"

My eyes stung as he looked across at me, a grey bushy beard with spectacles perched on the end of his nose giving him the look of an old studious professor, except this man was my psychiatrist - someone qualified to help me in my time of need. The tears slowly trickled down my cheeks, leaving trails of black mascara staining my perfectly made up face. His following words sounded so remote, just like they were being transported down from a faraway planet, tucked away in the outer galaxy.

"Maybe you could seek advice from the ladies fronting the cosmetic houses in chemists and department stores? How does your Mum feel about the way you look?"

The trickle of tears soon escalated into a stream and feeling embarrassed with my vulnerability, I bowed my head in shame. I watched as the teardrops fell onto my lap, turning my blue denim jeans where they landed a shade darker in colour. Feeling an instantaneous urge to stand up and scream my mood suddenly changed as I violently kicked away the chair I had been sitting on.

Looking down at the psychiatrist my distress and frustration at his criticisms turned to anger and the only two things coming between us was his note pad and a half filled mug of coffee. He looked up at me puzzled, as I wiped away the remaining tears from my cheeks with the sleeve of my red fluffy jumper. This rather plump, yet distinguished looking gentleman, whose eyes constantly seemed to be interrogating me over the rim of his spectacles, didn't seem to understand why I was so upset. I moved in a little closer, noticing a large shiny gold buckle desperately trying to make an appearance between his pristine white shirt and trouser waistband, whilst the remainder of the leather belt was presumably hidden beneath layers of excess fat around his midriff. Numerous half-opened packets of biscuits lined the shelf behind him, which seemed to suggest his obvious love of food and as he rested his arms across the dark wooden desk, I began to explode.

"How dare you talk about me or my mum in such a way? Who are you to tell me how I should look, or dress, and precisely what has this got to do with my illness?"

I began to shake as my rage reached a tipping point. Still screaming angrily at him I quickly picked up my belongings and without waiting for his response flew out of his surgery, back into the waiting room. The tears once again welled up in my eyes as I awkwardly wrestled with my coat, battling to pull my left arm through the appropriate sleeve, whilst at the same time trying to zip the main compartment of my handbag.

A friend, who had come along with me for support was sat waiting patiently for my appointment to finish, her head buried inside a lady's fashion magazine. I called out her name and she looked up at me in utter disbelief. There I was, looking an absolute mess, standing there with just my right hand in the sleeve of my coat, the contents of my handbag strewn all across the floor and my red face covered in make-up streak lines. How could I have possibly allowed this man to make me feel so bad and all because I didn't fit into his limited perception of the female role in society!

There was no doubt my appearance was a little eccentric. I stood out in a crowd, with curled, lacquered bleached blonde hair and a perfectly placed beauty spot resting on my cheekbone whenever I ventured out. It was also no coincidence either that the way I looked was heavily inspired by my childhood icon, the Hollywood movie star Marilyn Monroe, but whilst my parents cringed at many of the outfits I chose to wear, they barely ever got in my way. Oversized coats, the shortest miniskirts, six inch platforms and blood red lips, no matter how embarrassing my image may have got for them, they realised how I wished to express myself was my journey and not theirs.

"*My God Sharon, what's happened? I thought you were here to be helped, you look awful!*"

Neither of my parents could make this appointment and I had gladly accepted my friend's offer to accompany me. There was no reason to think the meeting with my psychiatrist would be any different to previous visits. It had always been the same trainee doctor, maybe still learning the skills, but she was lovely and seemed to understand exactly how I was feeling. It had been quite a shock to see her replacement that morning, however, it didn't take long to realise after preliminary introductions with the head of the department, my consultation with him was going to be a lot less empathic and dreadfully uncomfortable.

"*Sharon, are you okay?*"

My friend had already dropped the magazine she was reading, galloped over to me and was now busy picking up the contents of my handbag from the floor. I couldn't bring myself to discuss with her what had happened because my mind was racing, spinning, and I was hurting so much the psychological pain was excruciating. All I wanted to do was run away, run outside into the main road, hopefully in front of a bus. Find a place where no one knew me, somewhere I wouldn't be judged, a place where nothing mattered anymore, somewhere I could simply be myself without any disapproval. Looking back now, I will always be eternally grateful for my friend's company that day because if I had been on my own, I doubt I would have been here to tell the tale.

Later that day, over our teatime meal, I managed to convince Mum and Dad I had been given a clean bill of health and was therefore discharged from the clinic. They had been through so much during my illness, so to see the relief on their faces when I told them my fabricated story clarified to me that neither of them needed to know the reality. Besides, I was absolutely determined to prove the psychiatrist's theory had been based purely on his own personal bias and this was now my ultimate goal, whilst I also vowed and declared I would never return back to a clinic again.

CHAPTER 3
THE NEXT THIRTY YEARS

'With a jet set career, would fears disappear?
Would she be sophisticated like the rest?
And would men see what a catch she'd be
Being cultured and designer dressed?'

Looking back at my thirty years preceding 2010 can seem rather scary and it is sometimes hard to believe where the time has gone. The disoriented young woman beset, but yet in some ways encouraged by the words of a misguided psychiatrist. Thwarted by the man's ridiculous notions of how a female should behave, how she should look and what role she should play in society. Unknowingly rewinding and replaying over and over again in my mind his few cutting words during the consultation, consequently allowing his personal theories to be the dominating factor behind every decision I made.

Now, as a middle aged lady transformed reluctantly by the passing of time, I can look back on those years with fondness and appreciation, rather than regret. I have come to understand that although through my own weaknesses I may have often been misdirected down the longest, most difficult and sometimes treacherous roads to achieve my goals, the lessons I learned were palpable.

It was the factory where I was working at the time of my psychiatric appointments that became the initial platform from which I remoulded my life. I took the first scary steps, turning a dead end job into a career and for the next fourteen years worked my way up through the internal ranks, brushing aside any negative advice from people whose motives were not entirely for my benefit.

*'Don't let anyone say you can't, because you can,
Ignore what people say and make your plan,
Nothing is impossible
Don't falter, be unstoppable,
Don't let anyone say you can't, because you can!'*

It was a lengthy, rocky road from packer, onto supervising the company's distribution, to finally having my own desk in the marketing department and although often fraught with handicaps and disappointments, I can see now the challenges I faced have made me who I am today.

Jealousy and envy are widespread emotions within corporate organisations, which encourage competition and rivalry throughout a workforce, however, although these emotions are not confined behind company walls, it is where I first fell foul to their harmful effects. A few, who felt they had been overlooked by someone minor in years, who also believed I couldn't possibly match their intelligence simply because I was merely a factory girl, turned their venom into anger. Their gossip and spite hardly interfered with my work ethics, as I continued to work late into the evenings and weekends to ensure that not only the company targets were met, but more importantly my goal to prove my worth in society was accomplished. I have never been under any illusions about my own personal vendettas engineered by jealousy and envy, but through my recent mindfulness practices and meditation, I have come to realise although these feelings are perfectly normal, the danger stems from when we allow them to hang around for too long. These types of emotions can very quickly turn to rage and are soul destroying, not just for the injured parties caught up in the incensed behaviour, but for the vexed deliverers too.

Eventually their animosity began to cloud the working

atmosphere and this started to screw up my mind, until I started to argue with myself about the abilities I had to succeed in a professional environment. The results I had already achieved in my distribution role didn't seem to matter anymore, so one afternoon I took drastic measures, walked out of the dispatch office, through the company gates and headed home, leaving numerous tasks undone. Phone calls and meetings with the heads of the company eventually brought me back into their fold, but my actions only antagonised. Resentment grew stronger, the hostility worse, but the nightmare was eventually resolved when I successfully secured a promotion into the company's marketing department, leaving the malicious gossip behind me.

Working in a sales capacity, preferably on the road as a sales executive was my absolute intention and I do remember when clinching the marketing position being quizzed by the Managing Director about my motives. I had spoken to him a few months previous about my goal and I think he worried I saw the marketing position as a stepping stone to my dream career. I probably did, because a short while later, in 1994, I left the company to begin almost sixteen years doing exactly what I had set out to do. For the first eighteen months I was selling and merchandising chocolates, until I finally secured what I perceived to be the ultimate prize.

Throughout this time my love life was almost non-existent, but I never gave up, and constantly searched for someone who I considered to be the right man for me. As I progressed with my career the hunt turned to members of the opposite sex who I deemed appropriate to compliment my new role, so they were not only judged by their appearance, but by their status too.

My first and last marriage proposal took place at the tender age of eighteen and as I had only been dating the boy eight weeks, I quickly declined the offer. Since this time I can categorically say there has been no one who has truly loved me. Perhaps wined and dined me, encouraged my infatuation for them, even bedded me, but none were supportive, or a loyal friend. I don't blame any of these men because I seemed to constantly set myself up to fail. Chasing and grasping at potential partners, who would either run in the opposite direction after seeing the desperate look in my eyes, or flattered by the attention they would abuse the situation. I was a woman possessed, on a mission to prove that the Psychiatrist's theories were wrong.

It was during my short spell on the factory floor I met my best mate Marie. For thirty-five-years even though we are total opposites and our paths have taken each of us in completely different directions, the close friendship has weathered the test of time.

For a short while we lived together in rented accommodation, an upside down flat above 'Relate' marriage guidance. The rickety wooden staircase that led to the first floor living quarters resembled the steps leading from the lower cabin of a boat onto its deck and was certainly the accommodation's best feature. The two bedrooms were situated on the ground floor alongside the kitchen and bathroom, overlooking an extremely busy road leading out of the town centre. Most evenings our sleep would be interrupted by the noise of traffic, or police incidents, so it wasn't long before we moved out and into a slightly more upmarket abode.

A two bedroomed house, complete with garden and stone ornamental bird bath, which initially was barely visible because the lawn was so overgrown. We didn't stay there too long either, my Dad suddenly fell terribly ill and with my brother living in Norwich, I made the decision to move back home and help Mum with his care. Paying my half towards the bills and rent had started to become increasingly more difficult for me since starting my new job, so giving up my independence didn't take much persuading.

In my early thirties, I hadn't been long in my new sales role, but although the financial package offered to me included a brand new company car and exciting bonus prospects, I had also made the choice to take a small cut in salary. It seemed a small price to pay for the experience and training I would gain from a blue chip company. My spending and borrowing was probably relatively normal at the time, however, my desire to look good over the years had already made some deep impressions on my credit cards and I now needed to tighten my purse strings.

Marie and I parted ways after a few years sharing food bills, pot washing and home parties. Since this time we have fallen out, made friends, cried on each other's shoulders and shared our most intimate secrets, but most importantly through good times and bad times we have held on to a very special friendship. People come and go in our lives, this is reality, part of our journey, however, it doesn't stop the experience from being painfully sad sometimes. For various reasons we lose contact with others, maybe we change course, or perhaps their working patterns altar, but whatever the motive is, people disappear from our circle of connections.

As we make our way through life we invariably store memories of past events, experiences and moments, all of which can manipulate and hinder our future if we don't take control. It's the same with relationships too, and even though there are people we are probably glad to see the back of, who maybe didn't cut the mustard, or make the grade, every single bond, association, or connection is beneficial to our spiritual growth. If we only take time to pause and reflect, we can generally see the lessons we need to learn.

The most difficult situations, the toughest relationships are so often packaged with invaluable messages. I have experienced my fair share of both, but sadly through knee-jerk reactions I often failed to pause and jumped the red warning light. Patience helps to delay our response in times of exasperation or disapproval, gives a much broader perspective of the situation, helping to replace the negative emotions with compassion and forgiveness. Maybe this was the lesson I needed to learn, because I look back at the times I have regretfully exploded like an atom bomb, attacking unsuspecting victims, who I have deemed guilty of an injustice to me and it has never made the situation any better. Perhaps sometimes my perceptions were right, but lashing out without first taking a deep breath to think things through never made me feel good and I doubt it made the offender feel brilliant either. No one has to be a pushover and we shouldn't have to tolerate bad behaviour towards us either, but any pent-up frustrations that can ultimately turn to anger isn't good for our health.

Death is something we can't defer or avoid, it happens to every single one of us and when our departure from life finally arrives, it is the people we leave behind who feel the most pain. There is nothing more heart-breaking when someone we dearly love disappears from our network of connections because of their passing and I remember the first time I felt this wretched grief. We have lost family pets, this is always difficult at any age, but losing Grandma at thirteen was my first introduction to the inescapable sorrow. After Grandad passed away she didn't cope well on her own, so Dad, who was becoming increasingly more worried about her welfare, eventually encouraged her to stay with us. Grandma and I had grown immensely close in the year leading up to her death. She became my soul mate, a sounding board to discuss parent issues over spotty dysfunctional boyfriends. We had spent so much time together during her last months, it took quite some time for me to come to terms with the terrible void she left behind. I still remember Grandma with fondness today, her apron, hair nets, and towards the end her continual yearning to be with Grandad in the next life.

Once back home with Mum and Dad, the itch to increase my salary and status had me searching the back pages of the 'Grocer' retail magazine. It seemed inundated with job possibilities and now I had some blue chip sale training, I couldn't see there would be much difficulty in getting interviews. Besides, I wanted to buy my own home, but with very little in savings, the only solution was to improve my salary. Dad was feeling much better after recuperating from a life threatening operation, so for the time being there was some normality back in our family lives. It didn't take long before I made the switch from a Team Leader merchandising confectionary, to an Area Sales Manager selling travel accessories. With a bigger car, higher monthly income and much more bonus potential, the model life I had visualised for so long was almost complete.

In 1997 I bought my dream home, it seemed only fitting that after achieving the role of an independent female executive, I should acquire a property appropriate to the new-found status. It was largely borrowed money, however, this wasn't such a big deal at the time, as all the banks were crying out for first time buyers and only a small deposit was needed.

It baffles me how I managed to even scrape together the required deposit, but with the miniscule savings I had and a small loan from my parents, somehow I pulled it off. The bank was very quick to offer their assistance too, they not only granted me the mortgage, but also a loan against the house to buy furniture and white goods. Dad had been key in turning the two bedroomed semi-detached into a home and in no time it was decorated in all my favourite colours, adorned with pictures and soft furnishings congruent with my taste.

I had finally succeeded in getting everything I initially set out to achieve, so why did it still feel as though there was something missing. A jet set career woman dressed in pencil skirts and matching jackets with brief case in hand, new learned IT skills, monthly pay packets, company car and bonus payments, all now a reality and yet the downs still outweighed the ups. For thirty years I had been continually fighting, almost drowning in waves of highs and lows, but because I never truly learned how to stay afloat during complicated setbacks, the spells of happiness were short-lived.

"Why doesn't it feel like the perfect life I had dreamed it would be?" I couldn't stop asking myself the question over and over again. The answer was simple, however, I couldn't see it then. I never believed in myself, therefore I wasn't happy within, so I doubt it would have mattered how high I climbed up the corporate ladder, how big my house or car was, and how fancy my clothes were, nothing would ever have been good enough.

CHAPTER 4
THE FIRST SIGN

*'But the warning call will always come
in different ways and in surprises,
And every time it is ignored
It will try on new disguises.'*

Just a couple of years into my new role as a sales executive I believe I received my first warning call trying to encourage me to change the direction in which my life was heading. In high spirits, I had almost completed a two-hour journey from Derbyshire to Cheshire and was now driving along the last few miles stretch of the M56 motor-way.

Early Friday morning I was on my way to visit a client in Chester, who I now considered to be an extremely good friend. I had met so many wonderful people since starting out with the company, which helped to make the untimely morning wake up calls, long journeys and late nights much more bearable. I had quickly learned the reality of a middle class professional woman was not quite how I had envisaged it would be, but never the less, the position gave me freedom of choice in planning my days and the ability to work out the best strategies and approaches for meeting my targets.

Thoughts of the shop manager's usual fresh coffee on arrival started to tickle my taste buds. I could almost smell the aroma of the coffee beans under my nose as I indicated and manoeuvred into the middle lane of the motorway. I pondered whether to give Marie a call later that day as I began to overtake a couple of vehicles driving steadily on the inside lane. We generally kicked started our weekend at a country pub called 'The Fox and Goose', however, in a conversation a few days earlier we were undecided what to do. Now, the idea of a few glasses of wine to round up a particularly stressful week was starting to become increasingly appealing.

The motorway was fairly quiet, but this wasn't unusual for a Friday morning. I think most travelling business people scheduled their diaries to stay local, or work from home and reflecting on the events that followed, I maybe should have done the same that day.

A small van just ahead of me suddenly swerved erratically and within the blink of an eye the Toyota I was driving lost control. It all happened very quickly, a large chunk of metal fell from a lorry travelling in front of the van and when the driver saw the debris heading straight for his vehicle, he must have manoeuvred to avoid a collision. Unfortunately for me, because of his actions the van clipped the runaway junk, which sent it hurtling straight into and under my car.

Suddenly my Toyota seemed to have been possessed, taken over by the devil. The sounds from the horrendous clattering noises caused by the scrap metal entangling itself with the underbody of the car and the violent shaking within the vehicle was terrifying. In a mad panic to regain control, I frantically tightened my grip on the steering wheel, whilst continually slamming my foot hard onto the brake pedal. But deep in the pit of my churning stomach I knew - it was time to stop, there was nothing left that I could do. What seemed like hours must have only been seconds, but I do remember unexpectedly feeling peacefully calm, as I first released my foot from the brake pedal and then removed my hands from the steering wheel. I figured that whatever happened next was simply out of my control. Looking back, I see it as a perfect example of letting go of an external situation I had no power to change. I didn't know if I was going to die, be seriously injured, or come out of the accident totally unscathed, but something I will always remember is after making the decision to let it be, I no longer felt scared. *"Don't think I will be going to the Fox and Goose this evening after all!"* My last thoughts, as the car finally raced across the motorway towards a crash barrier on the hard shoulder.

I don't recall much about the final impact, however, the vehicle must have hit the barrier with such ferocity that it forced the car to spin around, so the front end was facing the motorway. The queues started to build as the vehicles began slowing down to witness my predicament and still in shock, I started to feel each of my body parts to make sure they were all intact. I realise how lucky I was to have emerged from the wrecked Toyota without a single blemish, but there were many factors in my favour on that day, which in my opinion helped to keep me alive. It was Friday, the motorway was quiet, no other vehicles were travelling near me as the car hurtled across two lanes, and I now believe my relaxed state at the time of the smash protected me from serious injury too.

I was on the phone to Mum and Dad, when both the front passenger and driver's doors flung open simultaneously. Suddenly peering into the car were two knights in shining armour, whose white vans I barely noticed had pulled up at either side of the car. For months I had cursed the infamous drivers of white vans for every infringement of the Highway Code and yet here they were, the first to my rescue. A squabble emerged between the pair of them as they each gave me their conflicting instructions on what I should do, so it was quite comforting when the police arrived to administer the situation. I was still sat traumatised in the driver's seat when one of the officers held out his hand to help me out of the car.

"Let's get you somewhere safe until the medics arrive to check you over."

Sitting in the back of a police car taking a standard breathalyser test was not something I would have conjured up doing that Friday morning, but at least I was still in one piece, which was more than could be said for the car I had been driving, it looked completely broken.

I had refused to go with either of the two ambulances when they arrived on the scene, instead asking if I could go with the Toyota and tow truck to the garage. My brother Paul lived close by and had made arrangements to leave work so that he could take me home. He collected me from the garage shortly after my arrival, but I don't think he was prepared for the extensive damage that had been done to the car. I later found out he had told my parents that after witnessing the state of the vehicle, he couldn't believe how lucky I had been to escape without any injuries.

Dad encouraged me to get checked out at the hospital and to make sure I went he offered to take me. We laughed heartily together on our way back to the car, discussing the unsightly neck brace I was made to wear whilst enforced to lay flat out on a trolley bed. It had been over twelve hours since the accident, but the hospital assured me they needed to take the necessary precautions for a neck or spinal injury. Thankfully I left the Accident & Emergency department that evening with a relatively clean bill of health.

I have always wanted to believe there is something, or someone watching over us, who knows more than we do, who understands why we are here and who takes care of us until they know it is our time to go. On that Spring morning in 1999, it definitely felt like there was an unexplained phenomenon with me in the car, sprinkling magic across its fateful path and cushioning me from harm, so the first warning sign could be given to hopefully redirect me down another path. Just one of numerous warning signs I chose to ignore over the next ten years.

Showering on a work day was generally a two-minute exercise due to time constraints, nevertheless, I tended to use those precious moments for indulgence with expensive skin care. The warm soapy water streamed from the showerhead, as I allowed it to wash over me, basking in the delights of my new coconut based body cream, and it was then I felt the alien mass on my right bust for the first time. I froze like a robot whilst the water persistently bounced from my lowered forehead, straight into the bath and because of its relentless contact, my saturated hair fell over my eyes. I couldn't believe the bad luck I was having, but all I could do was keep feeling the tainted area, hoping I had made a mistake.

My family were furious about the decision, but on the Monday after the accident I was back behind the wheel of my car and working. My thinking behind this was to dispel any driving fears that could have evolved from the incident, however, nothing, not even my health was going to get in the way of this endless pursuit for a career consumed with success and stature. I don't think the judgement call I made was a particularly wise one because a few months later I was seeing a specialist, after being diagnosed with delayed trauma. My decision never to see a psychiatrist again had also been tainted, but I consoled myself with the notion he was a councillor working on behalf of my insurance company, which in my eyes was something completely different. Jumping straight back into the saddle caused repercussions with my health that could most probably have been avoided, however, at the same time it helped with the compensation claim, being rewarded a few thousand pounds for my shock, ordeal and inconveniences.

I had only been given the all-clear by the councillor a few weeks previous. After evaluating me for any possible mental issues derived from the car crash he reckoned there was no permanent damage, assuring me the flash backs and nightmares would eventually be less frequent, until they stopped completely. So now this! I don't know how long I had been standing there with the water spilling over me, but feeling cold and shaky I finally stepped onto the bathroom mat, wrapping a warm towel around me. The sickening feeling when I found the abnormal lump on my breast that morning was numbing. I didn't go to work, but headed straight to my parents for advice. If there were two people I could count on for support and comfort, it was Mum and Dad.

Within six weeks I was diagnosed, treated and discharged from the hospital and I will never be able to praise the NHS enough for their competence during this time. Fortunately for me the outcome was a positive one, the screening was showing a non-malignant large cyst, which was drained instantly whilst I watched the procedure from a monitor by my bed.

Just turned forty, my life raced before me in the shower that morning, as I contemplated the many desires I still needed to bring about. The aspirations I hadn't yet accomplished, plans in need of executing and babies I still hoped to carry. The question of childbirth had badgered me for quite some time and whilst I sat with my doctor during the emergency appointment later that day, I quizzed her about her views on mid-life Motherhood.

"At what age do you think it becomes unsafe to carry a child?"

I desperately wanted a baby, but with no potential Father even on the horizon, pregnancy was looking bleak and now dubbed by the fears of my findings in the shower, it almost seemed like time was running out.

"Forty-five" was her answer, so after the car accident and cancer scare, I decided it was time to step up the search for prospective partners.

CHAPTER 5
150 MILES AWAY

*'Her Father's death was the hardest thing
In the year 2003,
The toughest blow, the biggest sting
The most painful memory!'*

Wednesday November 12th 2003 had been yet another exasperatingly busy working day in London. Each year around this time the company I worked for launched their new collection from a luxurious hotel in the capital and with only two days left in our rigorous schedule, I had mischievously coerced one of the team to take me out that evening.

"Let's split the week up and have that night out we keep promising ourselves." I suggested.

I had spotted a great play advertised in the West End and I reckoned a visit to the theatre, mixed with a little retail therapy and a bite to eat beforehand, was just the pick me up we both needed. Although part of a close-knit sales team, our friendship had developed into something quite special since I started out with the business in 1996. Most working days, we would call one another to check how things were. A sounding board for each other, musing over any problems with clients, orders, or even management.

"How about champagne in Selfridges too perhaps?" I asked excitedly.

He did not take much convincing, we had been threatening an evening out together for quite some time so the thought of spending a few hours away from the bosses, whose conversations seemed to revolve purely around the following year's targets, couldn't have been more tempting.

It was a few weeks prior to the company exhibition whilst surfing the internet I noticed an advertisement for the play, but it was the leading role that initially sparked my interest. An actor, who I had admired for a number of years was headlining the stage production and I remember daydreaming about how I managed to catch his attention from a front row seat, as he delivered his lines so perfectly. Captivated by his beautiful blue eyes, he then whisked me off my feet, held me tightly and delivered the one kiss that would change my life completely. It never occurred to me during this visualisation that he could possibly be married, however, the thoughts of finally finding true romance with someone, who was not only extremely talented, but looked delicious too seemed worth fantasising about. The search was still ongoing in finding my Mr Right, but sadly this was probably down to continually looking in all the wrong places. I purposely forgot to mention my obsession with the leading actor to my friend, so with his blessing the tickets were booked.

The company exhibition had gone on a lot later than we had anticipated, but although we were both extremely weary, we were also still determined to make the most of our evening together. With only a couple of hours to spare before the opening of the play, we stepped outside the hotel giggling and reminiscing about two very drunk customers, who seemed determined to stay until the last remaining bottle of wine was empty. Their order was quite substantial, so this compensated for the copious amounts of wine and bubbly they had consumed during the course of the day.

The taxi pulled up outside Selfridges and the almost too familiar adrenalin rush swept over me. I frantically searched inside my latest black designer handbag, pushing aside my hair lacquer, deodorant and an assortment of perfume bottles, until I could feel the Gucci purse purchased a few weeks earlier. With a sigh of relief, I quickly opened the card section, gently caressing a number of visa cards reassuringly with my thumb. Staring back at me was the exquisitely prestigious American Express card, which I had purposely placed on top of the selection. Plastic gave me an ability to spend lots of money and this somehow triggered an excitement, making me feel extra special, even if it was only for a short while. In a department store simply oozing with glamour, stardom and wealth, my six inch heels, tight fitted black dress, credit cards and faux fur jacket seemed to fit the bill perfectly.

We were extremely good mates and the laughter spilling out from one of Selfridges champagne bar's only helped to confirm this. Aperitifs washed down with a few glasses of Moet fuelled the giggling to fever pitch. It was so good to relax after such a hard day, but I needed to do some serious shopping before the theatre and I was also desperate to see the 'Agent Provocateur' lingerie department too.

His face was a picture whilst I browsed through the beautifully displayed underwear and still feeling the effects from the champagne and its bubbles, I teasingly held up an array of corsets and bras for a sign of approval. Red faced with embarrassment, he eventually walked away from the department pointing to his watch, whilst mouthing silently *"ten minutes only."*

The champagne had clearly gone straight to my head, so I was left alone to peruse the displays a little while longer and within seconds I was already trying on two matching sets of lingerie in the changing rooms.

"Why buy one set, when there is enough plastic in my purse for two."

My mouth watered with excitement as I watched the assistant wrap the pieces of lingerie perfectly in soft tissue, before dropping them into a stylishly decorated box. She looked up at me quoting the total cost of my purchases, her make-up looked flawless, blushed cheekbones and ruby red lipstick that matched pearly white teeth perfectly. I handed over my American Express card and she beamed a radiant smile. *"Is there anything else we can tempt you with today Madam?"*

I hurriedly scanned the department to check if there was something, anything that would shout out at me and entice me to buy, but all I could see was my friend, who had now returned to collect me and was standing at the edge of the department vigorously pointing to his watch again.

I am still not sure why I chose lingerie to purchase on that November evening in Selfridges. There was still no man in my life to impress, however, I am wondering if I may have read in one of the many self-help books I had purchased over the years that true happiness, contentment and confidence could only come from within. If this was the case I certainly don't think I had quite grasped the concept, convoluting what was probably a straightforward message to find inner peace. The idea I may have believed wearing glamorous underwear would help me create a life of dreams just makes me realise how much work really needed to be done inwardly. Perhaps the Agent Provocateur lingerie may have felt empowering underneath works suits and elegant party dresses, but apart from racking up another two hundred pounds on my next month's visa bill, I doubt there was little else to be gained.

My friend was now fully acquainted with my secret fascination for the leading actor and patiently endured my continual drooling each time the star looked out towards us from the stage. My dream though was merely a fantasy, but the night was perfect anyway. Sitting in front row seats allowed our brains to engage with the plot so much more, we seemed to be drawn onto the stage and into the play's unfolding storyline.

We enjoyed the show immensely, so after it had finished

we decided to bring the evening to a close with a glass of wine in a bar situated next door to the theatre. The obvious choice, not only to us, but the rest of the theatre goers too, looking at how busy the pub was. The only few remaining empty seats were ridiculously high stools and trying to get comfortable on one of them wearing a tight black dress and six inch heels was almost impossible. I had just managed to perch myself precariously by the side of my friend when I noticed the leading actor stroll past the window, clutching a garment carrier. I leapt from my stool pointing to the window and without waiting for my friend's response I ran out into the cold dark London Street. I couldn't see him initially, but then emerging from behind the back of a standing taxi, I noticed the familiar slim figure. Watching him drop his garment carrier into the boot, I ran as quickly as I possibly could in my high heels towards him. Slamming the lid shut, he turned and there I was - a pen in one hand, a programme in the other.

"The play was amazing this evening. Would you please sign my programme?"

My heart was pumping hard, racing fast, although I do think this was perhaps down to the unexpected running exercise rather than the excitement of meeting my idol. His long cream coloured rain coat suited his tall stature and whilst he autographed the front cover of the souvenir brochure he was delightfully sweet. Handing me back the pen and signed copy, he smiled, wishing me a pleasant evening.

"Maybe he wasn't to be my knight in shining armour after all."

I felt a little disappointed, but just like an excited child I ran back into the pub waving the autographed programme for my bewildered friend to see.

"My God Sharon, I was starting to wonder if you were

ever coming back."

He pushed the untouched glass of red wine towards me, just as my mobile phone suddenly lit up on the pub table and the unmistakable Madonna ring tone began to play. I was still trying to clamber back onto the barstool when I realised my brother's name appeared as the caller.

"Oh my God! It's my brother!"

I immediately handed the phone to my friend realising instantly this could only be bad news. It was gone eleven o' clock, Paul would not be phoning me if it wasn't something serious.

"Please take the call for me!"

He grabbed the phone from my hand immediately answering the call and my brother's words I can still remember today.

"Please can you organise a taxi to bring my sister home to Chesterfield immediately, her Father is dying."

"No that can't happen. I'm not there. I can't lose my best friend!" Totally oblivious to the attention I was drawing towards myself I began screaming loudly, whilst frantically pacing the floor trying to grasp what my brother had just said. Panic set in when I suddenly realised I was 150 miles away from home and as I clumsily gathered together my handbag with the signed programme, I bellowed to my friend to get off the phone so we could find a taxi quickly.

My friend took complete charge of the situation, which is something I will never be able to thank him for enough. He wasted no time in getting me speedily back to the hotel, he helped me pack my suitcase, and then put me in a cab for the long drive home to Chesterfield. How easily happiness can turn into despair, and that evening was a perfect example.

The taxi driver must have had a harrowingly difficult

journey along the M1 to the Derbyshire market town, because unusually for me I never spoke one single word. What he looked like, how old he was, what nationality - I have no recollections of the man who drove those 150 miles in the early hours of a November Thursday morning.

As the car sped along an almost deserted motorway, I gazed out through the passenger window mesmerised by the dancing night shadows and the reflections created by distant lights, trees and buildings as we passed them by. My mind drifted as I started to think about the rotten hand Dad had been dealt during his seventy-one years of life.

My brother and I were still fairly young when he was forced into early retirement from a painting and decorating trade, a proud man it almost crucified him. It was heart-breaking to realise that Dad's illnesses had finally won the battle, even though he had fought so hard to maintain the upper hand. Despite all this though he maintained his dignity and no matter how tough things got, he would not allow his self-worth, or optimism to be intimidated. Once he accepted his fate and whilst continuing his ongoing fight with the crippling disease rheumatoid arthritis, he braved new worlds, ones which he probably would never have dared to choose should the circumstances have been different. He was a wonderful Father, a perfect role model, who always declared there were others far worse off than himself, even during his most difficult days. So many times I would hear him say *"There is always someone worse off than you"* and I couldn't help smiling when I remembered the last time I bore witness to these words.

We had been to the football match together earlier in the afternoon, armed with our usual flask of tea with a bag of mixed sweets, we always enjoyed those few hours urging our local club to victory. Due to his illnesses Dad often looked frail for his years, but he was certainly in good spirits during the football game as we cheered on the team, drank warm tea and chomped our way through the sweetie goody bag. Each match we would take our turns in driving to the game, and this particular day was my turn behind the wheel. I had just locked up for the evening, after dropping him safely back home when the phone rang. Eager to change into my pyjamas I was already half way up the stairs and contemplated whether to let it ring. *"They'll leave a message or call back if it's urgent"* I mumbled to myself. I must have sensed the urgency because my instincts overturned my decision to ignore the call. I ran back down the stairs and picked up the receiver, only to hear my Mum's worried voice on the other end of the line. She sounded really frightened asking me if I would take Dad to the hospital so he could be checked over. Without any hesitation I grabbed my coat, handbag and car keys before heading straight back to my parents' home.

Within the hour Dad and I were walking through the automatic sliding doors into the A & E department. He turned to watch a young boy in a wheel chair pass by in the opposite direction. The little boy looked pale and thin. He was wearing a blue and white football hat, which I presumed was to cover the results of his chemotherapy treatment. Smiling jovially, he waved over to Dad, whilst a man in his early forties, probably his father steered the chair out through the hospital doors, back out into the car park. Close by their side, a smartly dressed blonde lady encouraged by the little boy's efforts also looked towards Dad, and trying to share his enthusiasm courageously raised a smile too. It was obvious she was struggling to keep up the pretence, but my Father in his usual kind, unwavering manner responded back to them both, replicating the same warm gestures the little boy had conveyed.

"There is always someone worse off than you." Dad whispered in my ear as we walked toward the check-in

desk. The sickening result for my Father that day was a stroke caused by clots haemorrhaging in his brain and although a relatively small one, it was the first of many that eventually took him away from us.

He had suffered as a child himself. At eleven years old he was rushed into hospital after unfortunately becoming the victim of a school boy prank that went terribly wrong. Two young lads who were throwing stones in the street decided to aim one of the pebbles straight at Dad, which sadly went into his eye. The surgeons tried their best to save it, but regrettably they couldn't, so from that day on he had to learn how to live with just the one. It wasn't easy being a young boy with a glass eye in school, yet he learned to live with the jibes and no matter how conscious he felt, he tried not to let it interfere with any of his dreams. He achieved so much regardless of the disability, even passing a gruelling heavy goods driving test later in his life. He wanted the licence so much, but mainly because he wanted to prove to himself he could overcome an obstacle deemed impossible with his affliction. At the same time, he believed it would encourage others suffering from physical abnormalities that nothing is impossible.

Coincidently, at this point in my thinking a huge transport lorry rattled past the taxi, bringing my thoughts to a halt and noticing familiar surroundings, I realised we had almost arrived at our destination.

As the taxi pulled up outside the hospital entrance, I called my brother instantly to let him know of our arrival and whilst I sat motionless in the back of the car waiting for him to collect me, my mind churned over the last few hours.

It was during the panic of throwing all my belongings into my case and travel bag, I found out it was already too late. My friend had already cleared the hotel wardrobe, bathroom and dressing table top of all my belongings in minutes, which was an absolute miracle because I never travelled light. All the hotel guests must have heard my screams when I realised Dad had already passed away. Sandy, my cousin had tried so hard to keep it from me during our telephone conversation, she simply didn't want my journey to be any more difficult than she knew it was going to be, but I inadvertently guessed, I sensed the sadness in her voice.

It was a bitterly cold early morning when I finally stepped out of the cab. My watch was barely visible in the dim light of the taxi, but it looked to be around 3.30am as my brother's familiar figure headed towards the vehicle. All I could think about was being with my Father, however, finally seeing him lying in the hospital bed, pale, still and without his cheeky grin, didn't make me feel any better. The reality set in, as I realised it hadn't all been a horrific nightmare, he wasn't going to wake up, and neither was I.

The man I loved so much was now in heaven, but yet I couldn't accept it was true, because I hadn't been given the chance to say a proper goodbye. It was only a few days previous he had waved me off from the doorstep of my parents' home, and I recalled with affection our last conversation on that day.

"Are you alright for money Sharon? Do you need any help?"

"Dad I'm fine." I replied, *"I'm away with work, so they will be looking after me. You be good until I get back home."*

Mum smiled lovingly as her husband turned and shuffled back into their bungalow.

"Take care darling and keep in touch." She blew a kiss, waved and watched me from the doorway, until my car turned the corner out of sight.

It was nearly a year ago since her worried phone call to

me, the unscheduled visit to the hospital after the football match and his shocking diagnosis. Since that time Dad had suffered a number of strokes, but his last one had been the most crippling leaving him partially paralyzed. After a period of time in a rehabilitating hospital his unyielding will to survive pulled him through once more and he was allowed home. It had been hard for my family to even consider the possibility that he may never return back to his soul mate, however, with planned coordinated home visits from the different medical units caring for him, Dad's quality of life was a little more improved. He had loathed being away from Mum, which wasn't helping his recovery.

Now here he was, lifeless in a hospital bed. I flung my arms around his frail cold body. He felt colder than the harsh November air that had greeted me a little earlier as I climbed out of the taxi. I chewed over our last few words again and again, until I eventually screamed at him through a river of tears.

"Why did you have to go Dad, when I wasn't with you and Mum? You promised me you would be good!"

The following weeks leading up to, during and after his funeral remain a complete blur to me, however, the one consolation during this time was knowing my best friend Marie understood because of her own loss. In a strange set of sad circumstances both her Father and Grandma died a couple of months before Dad, which not only brought our families closer together, but also helped to make the next few years seem a little more bearable for all of us.

CHAPTER 6
BARKING MAD

'Because amidst the drama, helping others would calm her
Allowing the darker days to become sunny,
Because the love in her heart, had been strong from the start
And for little kids she raised lots of money!'

"Perhaps if I organise a charity event it will take my mind off things a little," I suggested to Mum on the flight back home.

Mum and I were on the way back from a weekend trip to Dublin when I decided that organising a fund raising event would perhaps help me to overcome Dad's passing. He had done so much for charity over the years and I thought that perhaps whatever I accomplished could be in his honour.

Getting Mum on a plane to Ireland had almost been impossible. Shortly after my Father's death I finally managed to convince her we needed a holiday, but I couldn't quite stretch the persuasion to flying, so although she applied for her first passport at sixty-six, we took the slightly longer route and travelled by coach to Dover, joining a ferry crossing to Spain. We stayed in a small seaside resort near Barcelona and although it was a wonderful little place, unfortunately for Mum her introduction to the Mediterranean was accompanied with four days of torrential rain. Most of the week's excursions were cancelled, but it didn't dampen our spirits because for the first time since Dad had died we learned how to laugh and have some fun again.

Six months after he passed away an all too familiar feeling washed over me and I became extremely ill. Depression had reared its ugly head once more, but even though I tried so hard to combat it, eventually the sickness dragged me kicking and screaming into the pits of hell. I isolated myself from family and friends, refused to go to work, because the trauma of facing people felt far too overwhelming. Finally, the doctor signed me off sick, his reason being a delayed trauma from my Father's death, so for almost eight weeks I barely had contact with anyone, cried solidly for days at a time and grieved. It certainly wasn't the first time I had been struck down with this type of mental illness, but the prescription for anti-depressants was definitely something new. My first introduction to Prozac medication, which was hopefully going to assist me in coming to terms with Dad's death. Since his funeral I had been struggling inwardly, trying to stay strong for Mum. My brother Paul was now married, living and working in Liverpool, however, although he had been a tower of strength during the time of the funeral, he couldn't watch over her in the way I could.

Feeling almost myself again, I decided it was time for me to get back into my working role, but before doing that I knew I desperately needed a short holiday, a change of scenery, so I discussed with Mum my intention to get away for a few days. I had scoured the internet for some favourable deals, thinking maybe a European city break would probably be the best option, however, Mum didn't seem too happy. She wasn't completely sure I had recovered enough to be travelling alone and with a concerned look on her face asked if she could accompany me.

"Mum, I will be extremely limited where I can go, because you will not fly!" I responded to her.

"Book something and just for you I will fly, but can we make it a short journey?" she replied hesitantly. And so before Mum could change her mind, our trip to Dublin was booked.

Mum squeezed my hand tightly as the plane lifted off into the air for our forty-minute flight. Her first experience in the sky wasn't to be the last, but she was exceptionally brave during her initial flight, though noticeably relieved when we touched down in Dublin's airport. It wasn't just the thoughts of flying which initially scared her, she had also been worried about the traumas of being a disabled passenger.

Mum had suffered quite a severe stroke in her early fifties, mainly due to exhaustion and stress. Coping with Dad's illnesses whilst maintaining a full-time job triggered the awful attack, but through her sheer determination she almost made a full recovery. Sadly, Mum was left with one disability. Unfortunately, the stroke had damaged a part of the brain controlling her balance. She had learned to master the handicap in the surrounds of her home, but in order to maintain an independent lifestyle with full mobility, Mum needed the assistance of a tri walker when out and about. The worries about her affliction being a hindrance were totally unfounded, since both the airport staff and flight crew were extraordinarily considerate. For weeks after, she relayed enthusiastically to friends about her conversation with the pilot as she waited for assistance from the plane. I truly believe Mum thought it was part of the hospitality package.

The dismal weather followed Mum and I once more on our travels, which was more of an inconvenience to me, rather than a disappointment. I had been suffering from a skin irritation brought about by stress and this was particularly sore around my eyes. Forced into wearing sunglasses under dark clouds and rain made me feel decidedly silly, however, the conspicuous looks I received from passers-by as they tried to figure out my reasons for going incognito was quite amusing. The Irish certainly know how to treat their guests though, and the Dubliners showered Mum and I with generosity during our visit to their beautiful country, making the weekend highly enjoyable.

Mum was certainly right about me not being completely healed, so although I returned back to work after our short break to Ireland, things were not as they seemed. The rosy picture I was once again painting about my life to other people couldn't be further from the truth. There was something far more sinister going on inside me and until this was dealt with my short periods of perceived happiness would only ever be temporary. The loathing I had for myself was incomprehensible, hatred I had coveted and nursed since being a young woman.

It wasn't the first time I had considered the notion of a fundraiser, because although the fright of my major car accident in the spring of 1999 didn't encourage me to make any drastic life changes, I did make a decision to give something back to society. If I had learned one thing, it was the realisation of how vulnerable we all are and how easily a story can have a completely different ending. Lives are changed in a matter of seconds, in ways we perhaps would never have imagined, through circumstances that can administer a devastating effect on our future. I reckoned being thankful for my narrow escape wasn't enough, so I set about organising my first ever charity event, raising funds for a national children's charity. I called upon Glenn, my friend and lead singer from the band Squeeze, to help me out. He agreed to do a solo acoustic gig in-between the band's tour dates supporting Blondie, and together on November 24th 1999 we raised a substantial amount of money for a worthy cause. The sense of achievement from the event's success far outweighed any euphoria from reaching work related targets, but oddly enough, I never felt compelled to do any more fundraisers until the idea struck once again on the plane back home from Dublin.

My second charity event took place on May 12th 2005 and from this time, until February 11th 2010 I organised three more, all of which raised a total sum of twenty thousand pounds for disadvantaged children. A strange few years, because although in one area of my life I was obviously ridiculously unhappy, spending a vast amount of money trying to recompense for troubled emotions, in another area of my life I was feeling extremely fulfilled, helping to raise a huge quantity of money for vulnerable kids. Never did the two intertwine, I was almost living a dual life, not quite Jekyll and Hyde, but I definitely had a thorny alter ego that was certainly a more dominant player, overshadowing my true nature.

The decision to rekindle my fundraising again was not only to help me overcome the pain of losing Dad, but to also continue where he left off. He loved helping others, however, he also enjoyed the stage, which is why he encouraged Mum to publically share her beautiful singing voice. Dad had bags of personality and this enabled him to mix with all types of people, whatever their class or stature. At the same time his engaging presence and infectious wit made it incredibly easy for him to captivate an audience, so for a number of years both my parents worked in the entertainment business. He formed a stage act called Kevin's Kabaret, which had them performing across England's working men's clubs circuit, but although a spring board for Mum's semi-professional singing career, it was also a fundraising quartet consisting of himself, a compere/comedian, his magician friend and wife assistant too. I feel fortunate to have been blessed with many of Dad's attributes. Inheriting his desire to help, his confidence to connect with others, but most of all his resilience when things got tough, all these qualities have assisted me in making each fundraiser a success.

It was early 2004 when I was first introduced to

Rosemary and I don't think she will mind me saying her first thoughts may have been something like, *"She is barking mad!"* I sat in the hotel lounge dressed in my favourite jeans, deliberately ripped across both knees, with frayed bottoms that rested upon my recently purchased winkle-picker red ankle boots. Bleached blonde curls spilled around the sides of a grey cloth cap, which I had placed neatly on top of my head to cleverly hide the hair's dark roots beginning to show through. A pink fluorescent writing pad lay on the table in front of me. It contained lots of my scribbled ideas, concepts that I hoped would assist me in successfully selling in the charity event's proposal during our meeting.

The obvious questions were fired back at me after I excitedly divulged my thoughts about a 'Celebrity Golf Day.' *"Can you play golf?" "Do you know any local celebrities who play golf?"* My answer to both was a resounding *"No"* and Rosemary, who was introduced to me by the charity's appeals manager suddenly gave me a discerning look. She and her husband were keen golfers; members of a prestigious golf club, both accustomed to taking part in charity golf tournaments. I could understand her concerns with my suggestions after hearing my response, but I knew I could do it and it didn't take me long before I had convinced Rosemary I could do it too.

Over the next two consecutive years my wild ideas jotted down in the pink notebook became a reality. With the help of Rosemary and a key number of volunteers, we held two very successful celebrity golf days, raising over £8000. The latter one in 2006 was made even more special, when Rosemary, who had now become a very dear friend, suggested we should hold the event in my Father's name. 'The Kevin Bull Memorial Golf Day' not only headlined our media advertising, flyers and tickets, but was engraved on the winner's trophy too. My dream had finally come true, a fundraiser officially and publicly held in my Dad's honour.

Sometimes it became extremely difficult trying to combine my full-time position as a sales executive with my part-time role as a volunteer, so I would often work into the early hours emailing local sports heroes and celebrities. Countless requests to take part in the contest, or donate prizes for the raffle were sent out, there was no one I considered unapproachable, neither was there anything that phased me. I seemed to gain a deep satisfaction from achieving results which others considered to be impossible and sometimes the doubters were right, but more often than not I was victorious in proving them wrong. This attitude hasn't changed today, however, the happiness I gleaned from my sense of purpose during this time was nothing more than phenomenal. I almost wanted to give the project my full divided attention, often feeling that my paid employment was getting in the way. Somehow though, I managed to make it work, until eventually I sadly paid the price and exhaustion, coupled with my other underlying issues put a strain on my wellbeing.

Plans for a further golf day in 2007 were already being talked about, its success had gained credence with the golf club where the event was held, but after the triumph of Dad's memorial competition I decided it was time to take a well-earned rest. I had pledged to bring the fundraiser back in 2008, however, the company I worked for had diversified into new markets and with increased responsibilities in my working role, there seemed little time for anything else.

My desire to be of service to others was so easily superseded by the urgency to be looked upon as a successful, affluent career woman. I listened to my ego far more than I listened to my heart, but yet in both body and soul I was far more uplifted when the goals I set for myself were in place to help make a difference for others. Working through my to-do list was never a chore for any one of the charity events, in fact even during the toughest times it was an absolute joy. If I was taking positive steps to reach a fundraiser's target, I found my attentions became so focused on the mission ahead that my own issues during this time seemed a lot less important. Helping others is one of the keys to true happiness and the amusing thing is I sampled my true vocation on a number of occasions, failing every single time to recognise how fulfilled I was during these spasmodic periods in my life.

CHAPTER 7
THE BUTTERFLY SYMBOL

'Steer me and guide me
Let my life flow,
In trusting awareness
Knowing when to let go.'

I have never remembered much about Dad's funeral; the date is no longer registered in my mind's diary of past events. A few strange anomalies on the day, for instance the lady who attended the wake, spoke to everyone, enjoyed the food, but when I asked who she was, no one knew. I found out at a later date she was a regular gate crasher at funerals. Apparently there are people who scan the church notice boards for the times and dates of funeral services so they can attend. Perhaps it's through loneliness, or the chance of free buffet food, whichever, it seems an extremely desperate pastime wanting to partake in such sad events.

I neither have memories of the readings, or my Father's eulogy, just the final piece of music 'Wind Beneath My Wings' by Bette Midler, who alongside Dusty Springfield and Petula Clarke ranked as one of Dad's all-time favourite singers.

The Priest's sermon at the crematorium is the only other recollection I have from that day. An especially warm-hearted, caring man, who seemed so different to the men of the cloth I had been used to as a child. Just after Dad passed away he told Mum the gates of heaven would always be open to her, or anyone else whose choice was to live a kind, loving and charitable life. Finally, a priest that made sense, who considered everyone to be equal regardless of money, stature, or religion. Mum wasn't a Catholic, but this didn't seem to matter to him, unlike before when I was growing up and the parish priest would continually badger her, telling Mum it was probably better for the children's upbringing if she also practised Catholicism.

I had been a stray from the church for many years, but had returned for a short period of time just after Dad's first slight stroke. The reason was purely because of the love for my Father, I knew this would make him happy. Don't get me wrong I believe in Jesus, perhaps more than I ever have, however, I have a problem with some of the pompous attitudes and man-made adaptations of religion, so I much prefer to practise my own personal type of faith. Learning from my mistakes, trying to forgive and be a much kinder person is not something I feel can be confined to a one-hour service on a Sunday morning, for me it is a full-time commitment, one which I am trying my best to maintain, but feel assured if I ever slip I will be allowed to try again and again until I get things right.

It makes me feel immensely sad when I see media footage of heads of countries, some of the most powerful men and women in the world, who have the capability to make changes that would see less poverty, abuse, illness, inequality, war, hatred and environmental catastrophes walk into holy places to spend an hour with God. A God, who I doubt would be in support of some of the decisions made by leaders across our planet today, so I can only assume this one hour a week must be simply to ease a conscience, hoping any sins will be forgiven when it is their time to leave this world behind them. My childhood theories with the 'Fancy Hats Brigade' hypothesis doesn't seem to have changed much at all and whilst I realise there are many good people across all religions, I also feel there are a few who choose to pick out the bits from prophesies that suit in order to justify their rules, unjust laws, wrongful decisions and selfish life styles.

My Father's face lit up when I walked into 8.00am mass unexpectedly one Sunday morning. I sat down beside him and his face was a picture of happiness. It was so obvious it meant the world to him for his daughter to be with him that day. He asked me if I would go to confession and make my return to the faith complete, so the following Saturday I went along with him extremely nervous, but satisfied to take on board his idea.

It had been an awfully long time since I had genuflected in the confessional box saying *"bless me Father for I have sinned"* and to be honest I probably should have written a list, because remembering every transgression over my non-practising years was going to be ridiculously difficult. Dad went in before me and alarmingly whispered in my ear as our paths crossed to and from the confessional box. *"Don't worry I have told the priest all about you, he'll be lenient so don't worry you will be fine."* The whole idea of being anonymous to the Holy Father had just been blown out of the window by Dad's selfless act for his daughter. But this was a priest who listened to my account of years away from the church, yet only wanted to welcome me back with open arms without lecture, or judgement, a priest who took Mum under his wing in her time of sorrow and the priest who read out the unforgettable sermon in the crematorium at Dad's funeral.

"Remember your loved ones are always with you, they may not be seen in body, but their spirit will always remain. Recognise the symbols they send to let you know of their presence. For example, if you see a butterfly at a poignant moment be assured this is a sign your passed loved ones are with you."

Three years after my Father's death a ray of light shone over our family when my gorgeous nephew Jude Anthony

Bull was born on May 2nd 2006. My brother's wife Joanne gave birth to a beautiful cute baby boy, who since this time has brought so much joy into all our lives. Most Aunties and Grandparents believe the children in their family are the best, but without a shadow of a doubt Jude certainly was to both Mum and I. Since being a toddler I have constantly joked with him telling him he is my favourite nephew and his unequivocal response is always the same, "I'm *your only nephew Aunty Sharon."*

It was the day of my nephew's christening when what I can only describe as a miracle occurred and the priest's sermon from my Father's funeral came to life. It was a warm summer's day and a delightful atmosphere nestled within the church, as many smiling, happy faces joined Jude's Mum and Dad in welcoming their son into the catholic faith. I was more than overjoyed at having been chosen to be a Godparent, realising that this responsibility was probably the nearest I would get to having my own child.

Halfway through the service Mum and I watched in amazement as a butterfly floated through an open doorway near the altar. The priest was just about to anoint my Godson's forehead when it began circling above family and friends invited to the ceremony. We turned to each other, obviously both recalling the words said in the sermon at Dad's funeral. As the butterfly continued to flutter around all the guests we burst into tears of joy, tinged only by a little sadness and I whispered under my breath, *"Love you Dad and so glad you have come to see your Grandson on his special day."*

Miracles happen every day of our lives, however, we don't seem to recognise them unless it's something we feel is an absolute life changer, like winning the lottery, but yet the birth of every living being is a miracle, no matter how small, or how irrelevant we may think they are in the web of life.

Dad taught me on a number of occasions the significant importance of other living creature's lives, but it was hard for anyone to believe our family story of the pet gold fish. Dad saved countless birds and mice from the claws of our pet cats, then reared them back to full health in the safety of the garage, however, when he gave our pet goldfish, who we had unequivocally named Goldie the kiss of life, this was a tale definitely to be repeated time and time again. We had been watching the pet fish float listlessly on his side in the bowl for quite some time. Realising he was probably dying my brother and I were becoming increasingly upset, but Dad wouldn't give up on Goldie that easily. He pulled him out of the water and started gently giving him the kiss of life whilst tenderly massaging his little wet body. To this day, I am not sure if it was a stroke of luck, or if Dad did manage to resuscitate Goldie, but it seemed to work and he lived for quite some time after.

Undoubtedly, as children the behaviours of our parents must have a far reaching effect in shaping what we become and how we feel as we get older, so I am certain Dad's show of kindness towards other living beings must have definitely rubbed off on me.

One thing I am absolutely certain of though, and that is my adoration of butterflies has increased tenfold since the day of Jude's christening.

CHAPTER 8
TRYING TO BUY HAPPINESS!

*'She'd often shop until she'd drop
It helped to lift her mood,
And with each designer dress she bought
She hoped she would be wooed.'*

Marie and I were sitting huddled together in our winter pyjamas on my dark green sofa. An icy cold January evening, we had pulled all the settee's scatter cushions around us, whilst we scoured the internet for relatively cheap hotel deals.

"More wine Marie?" I suggested, removing the laptop from my knee.

"London would be perfect; don't you think?" I shouted from the kitchen opening our second bottle of red Shiraz.

"We could travel down first class on the train. Mums would love that!"

I had arrived back into the lounge with our glasses half full once more.

"And we could take them to a show?" I continued.

I was already getting excited at the prospect of using the extra credit issued on one of my visa cards. Over the past year I had been finding things a little more difficult financially. My monthly salary was taking a beating from the repayments of three credit cards, an American Express card and the mortgage, but for now there was a silver lining and I was itching to start spending again.

Both Marie and I knew that Mum and Margaret (Marie's Mum) were both going through an incredibly difficult time. Coming to terms with the loss of their partners couldn't have been easy, so we thought by taking them on a short break together this would help distract them from their sorrow for a few days. London became the first of a number of trips we booked for the four of us and it was wonderful to see the pair of them smiling, enjoying their lives once more.

Our weekend jaunt to the Capital finally arrived and having enjoyed first class privileges on the train down to the city, we were all feeling extremely relaxed on our arrival into St Pancras. The station was buzzing with atmosphere, which couldn't fail to conjure up huge amounts of excitement and stepping from the train we chatted eagerly about our plans for the next few days. We giggled hilariously whilst we weaved our way through the hustle and bustle, following Mum's lead as she tactically manoeuvred her wheeled tri walker to gain access through the crowds. From years of experience she had learned how to use the walking aid to her advantage and it wasn't long before we reached the taxi rank.

After settling into the hotel, we decided a trip down Oxford Street would be the perfect start to our weekend break. We had already booked to see 'The Lion King' that evening, with a unanimous vote given for a Sunday visit to Covent Garden.

Shopping was an easy pastime for me, therefore it didn't take long before we had accumulated numerous high street carrier bags, each containing various brands of clothing, make-up and perfume. As we drifted in and out of the various department stores our legs began to feel the pace, so we decided to find somewhere to rest our legs.

Weary from too much walking and the weight of the bags, we strolled through Soho searching for a bistro with a menu to whet our appetites. Mums were busy chatting to one another a few yards behind Marie and myself, neither had noticed the scruffy looking elderly man heading in their direction. He strolled closer towards the nattering pair dressed in dirty trousers and a raincoat that was probably bought in cream, but was now miscoloured through a multitude of deeply ingrained stains. His trouser legs were clearly far too short for him, barely covering his shins and I wondered if they had perhaps been given away to charity after a washing day shrinkage disaster. He wore a pair of frayed burgundy braces over a worn out shirt, both looked like they had seen better days, yet both were proudly on display, because his raincoat no longer had any buttons. They were still oblivious to his presence as he stopped by them, but this was all about to change. With a disgusting leer across his face, he cocked his leg as far as it would go and proudly broke wind. Margaret and Mum were left flabbergasted, whilst he continued on his way. The noise had bellowed loudly from his lower region, rattling across the street and filtering into people's conversations as they sat enjoying drinks outside a pub. Heads automatically turned towards Mum and Margaret, because by this time the real culprit had disappeared.

Our bellies ached with laughter, as we repeatedly recalled the scene long into the evening, however, this was just the first of so many fun experiences we would share together. Memorable adventures, which not only temporarily blocked out my heartache, sadness and pain, but hopefully did the same for Mum, Margaret and Marie too.

Over the next couple of years, I booked numerous holidays, including City breaks and cruises with Mum, Marie and Margaret. There was never any expense spared through an inbuilt need I had for everything to be perfect, but particularly after Dad died, this crusade to endorse happiness for myself and everyone else became undeniably worse. A mission to accomplish joyfulness within others is a wonderful campaign, unfortunately though at this particular time the only way I could seem to see of raising smiles was by spending money lavishly. I would secretly search and book added extras for our holidays - better cabins, more baggage allowance and four star hotels. I lavished myself with fancy dresses, so that with each holiday booked my suitcase would be bursting at the zipper seams with extravagant items of clothing. My mind was still far away from understanding true happiness and until the root cause behind all the squandering was fixed, the never-ending splurges were just papering over the cracks, getting me deeper and deeper into debt.

I am often asked why the people closest to me couldn't see my spending was getting out of control and my answer to this is twofold. Firstly, at the height of my spending we were all preoccupied with our own personal grief, however, secondly, I was also an extremely good story teller - no one would have believed I was racking up so much debt.

It is often said money alone cannot buy happiness and when I look back over the years at my relentless squandering, assuming it would automatically help me to override many personal issues, I wholeheartedly agree. How often do we use external pleasures as a comfort blanket, hoping to resolve problems that ultimately we can only vanquish ourselves? Money is a useful source, one which we cannot live without, because it fuels the world we live in today and is necessary for our basic comforts, but whilst I hate to advocate it as being the route of all evil, so often it can be through misuse.

Our desperation to cling onto unloving relationships, our ongoing grasping of material things seems to derive from the ideology that superficial sources are intrinsic to a perfect life, however, unless we are at peace with ourselves inwardly this is a fallacy, which strips us of our true essence. Using my own personal delusions as examples in this book is surely testament to the fact that happiness reliant on anything, or anyone else is treading on shaky ground. Life can never be a continual bed of roses, but if we can find a way of loving ourselves for who we truly are today, not tomorrow, or in two months' time when we have lost weight, found a partner, or bought the perfect house, then even under the most punishing times, complications would be so much easier to endure.

I misconstrued happiness with status, believing the more I had, or was seen to have would be influential in pertaining love, admiration and friendships. I frantically wanted to be respected, craved for people to believe in me, to see me as a confident and vivacious woman, yet I didn't even believe it myself. The notion we need other people to approve who we are, holding them responsible for our contentment is the reason why we are so often let down.

"No man will marry you looking like that; men don't marry women like you!"

I had made these words the dogma of my life and because of this they have been the cause of many regretful actions, anger, frustrations and deluded misinterpretations. There is no denying I foolishly cherished my credit cards, saw them as gifts from heaven when they dropped through the letter box and used them to compensate for the emptiness I was feeling within. The question I needed to ask myself was why I saw shopping as the antidote for every trauma, dilemma and predicament, particularly when it was no longer making me feel jubilant, even for a short time. Those moments of elation, the adrenalin rush after making purchases were starting to be replaced with a physical sickness at the amount of money I had spent. Visits to the High Street in a working capacity were not helping the growing addiction either, making it all too easy to open my purse. A continual vicious circle of compulsive spending, followed by remorseful regret.

In 2008 I was delivered yet another major warning sign

when the financial rug was finally pulled from under my feet. It was the continual threatening phone calls from my creditors and months of sleepless nights which gave me no other option but to sell my beautiful home, throw away the cards and consolidate my £50,000 debt. The spending party was well and truly over.

I moved into rented accommodation, however, rather than be truthful about the situation, I preferred to play on the fact that a three bedroomed house would give me more space for visitors, rather than admit I could no longer afford the mortgage payments, alongside my loans, bills and credit card payments.

Ridiculous as this may seem, I had also started discussing fostering a child with a government agency, so this gave me another valid reason for requiring extra space within my home. I had a genuine desire to be part of a troubled infant's life, after being under no illusions I was well past the doctor's advised deadline for mothering a child of my own. The maternal instinct lay heavy on my heart, but although my intentions were honourable, I have no idea how I thought I could carry the application through with so much debt around my neck. It wasn't until I had passed the police checks and sailed through the first half of my interviews, I finally acknowledged how farcical the situation was, stopping the process going any further with the agency.

Once I had settled into my new home I began to look at the different options available to me for consolidating my debt. Although bankruptcy was one of the alternatives, I came to the conclusion that this would be a coward's way out. I felt I needed to learn some lessons in money management, so I arranged with a financial company to take out their IVA payment plan. For a little while life seemed to regain some normality, creditors were no longer allowed to call me and although I was having to live under a very strict monetary budget, I was encouraged at how easily I adapted to a life without access to credit cards and bank loans.

'UK in recession as economy slides!' This was the media's headline news in January 2009. Unemployment began rising at an alarming rate, high street sales had taken a frightening downturn and the stress at work became unbearable. The sales team I had worked with for thirteen years started to lose their spirit, but worse than this, after taking the extreme measures of selling my home to realign my life, I was about to find out that things were going to get a whole lot worse.

It was autumn 2009, the nights were drawing in, leaves were falling from the trees and my territory had been extended to cover the North East of England. My journeys were becoming unreasonably long, my working days dreadfully tiresome, but most of all I was feeling increasingly frustrated with the little time I had left for personal pursuits. The job had also started to lose its flavour, because over the past twelve months filling in spreadsheets for the new Sales Manager seemed to take precedence. Due to his never ending list of administration requests and to ensure I kept up with his demands, working on my laptop for hours in the evening after a prolonged drive home became more and more regular. I was constantly feeling under pressure, highly stressed and agitated through mixing late nights with early morning starts and this was beginning to put a strain on my wellbeing.

Knowing I had a long day ahead of me, I set off for Newcastle especially early. Having secured a substantial amount of business with a small high street chain, I wanted to be sure the merchandising was done correctly to encourage sales, so I planned to visit all four stores and help set up the displays. It was whilst I was hoisting my overloaded business bag from the car's back seat, I accidentally slammed my head into one of the steel girders of the multi-story car park. The pain was excruciating and seemed to flash from the back of my head through to my forehead. Feeling dizzy, but at the same time worried about getting to my first appointment on time, I simply rubbed the area that had received the blow, locked the car and headed off to my meeting.

After the knock to my head, a continual stabbing pain remained with me, but never once did I consider it to be connected with my accident earlier in the car park. A few hours later I was overcome with nausea, however, I simply put it down to exhaustion, being more frustrated by the inconvenience it was causing to my scheduled plans. I decided to take an early lunch break in the store's restaurant, hoping perhaps a bite to eat would help to reduce the constant pounding, but I didn't even manage one spoonful from the bowl of vegetable soup purchased.

The next two stores were both situated in retail parks on the outskirts of the city centre, so determined to continue with my day's work I bought a packet of painkillers. I hoped that by taking a couple of these tablets, this would help to reduce the dreadful headache enough for me to continue with my day. After a couple of hours there didn't appear to be any improvement at all, but much worse than this, whilst I was working on one of the merchandising stands within the store my legs began to give way. This was when I eventually realised there had to be something dreadfully wrong and whatever the cause, it definitely looked as though it could be a little bit more sinister than just a tension headache. Still very unsteady on my feet, with the head pains now almost unbearable, I made my excuses to leave early and set off for what was to be one of my longest and most harrowing journey's home.

I'm not sure how I managed to stay focused for two and

half hours behind the wheel of my car, but without every window open to keep me alert, I really do doubt I would have made it home. As darkness descended, the lighting from the roadside lamps alongside the A1 motorway conflicted with my vision, putting an extra strain on my driving ability. I battled with the elements for over 150 minutes as the cold air streamed from the open windows into my Toyota, and to say I am eternally grateful for arriving home safely that evening is not an understatement.

I didn't want to worry Mum when I got back, thinking perhaps a good night's sleep would cure whatever it was that seemed to be ailing me. After taking a couple more painkillers I hit the sheets, however, even though I was feeling completely drained I hardly shut my eyes. The severity of the headache never diminished, so the next morning after telling Mum about the previous day's events she insisted we paid the hospital a visit. She couldn't believe how ill I looked when I called to collect her, still, this was hardly surprising as the hospital doctor diagnosed me of having a severe concussion. He assumed it was triggered by a head injury sustained from the car park incident, but as if that wasn't scary enough, he also told me my decision to drive home the evening before and leave being checked out with the emergency department until the following day could have had serious consequences. He signed me off sick from work, telling me under no circumstances should I be driving long distances over the next few days, however, within a week I was back behind the wheel of my car northward bound.

Once again another warning sign unheeded, although shortly after I returned back to work things began to go horribly wrong. The final warning sign unbeknown to me was just around the corner and this time it was complete with alarm bells, red flags and danger signs, so there was no way it could be ignored. Time was running out because the road I insisted on taking was now becoming perilous for my health.

After a gruelling last quarter trying to meet the company's increasing target demands, whilst at the same time fighting off anxiety caused by both professional and personal pressures, I finally came to the conclusion to take a redundancy package offered to me by the company. My decision to do this wasn't really congruent with the way my role had developed either, as during the previous eighteen months, even amidst my depression, the country's recession and the new sales manager's aggression, there was an element of the business I had still enjoyed. Through the development of a number of new accounts I achieved the company's 2009 targets for business development, but moving goal posts and unscrupulous decisions made by the recently appointed boss, wasn't my idea of a perfect working environment. He seemed to have declared war on his inherited team, and so with a heavy heart I left the business in March 2010.

CHAPTER 9
THE LAST FEW HOURS

'So Prozac and drink replaced the spending
It helped to ease the pain,
And mixed with pizza, chocolate, crisps
The extra pounds she'd gain!'

Up until February 2010 when the event took place, my distressed mind had taken some solace from a charity cabaret event I had been organising with a group of volunteers. Once again the fundraiser was for disadvantaged children and somehow amidst all the chaos in my life, with the help of some wonderful friends we managed to raise a substantial amount of money. Recruited through the internet, artists from across the UK descended on one of the oldest theatres in my home town to perform for the cause. I think this was when I first realised the power social media had in helping to promote, but I doubt at that time I would have ever suspected it would play such an important role in a future business.

It wasn't long after the euphoria of the fundraiser's success my employment ceased, and for the first couple of months it almost felt as though I had been given an extended holiday. Since being a teenager I had always paid my taxes having never been without work, or taken any career breaks, so for a short period of time not being governed by early morning alarm calls seemed rather liberating.

In early May I decided to spend a few days away relaxing and visiting work colleagues who I hadn't seen in over six months. After almost three months trying to work out unsolvable solutions with company directors, accepting the redundancy in March and finally closing the door was a weight of my shoulder, so for a short period of time I was almost back to myself again. I boarded the 11.39 East Midland train bound for London St Pancras International, my destinations, Hastings, back to the Capital and then into Leicester on my homeward bound journey. Sat in a very busy carriage on the first leg of my journey, memories came flooding back as I recalled my last business visit to the capital. Sipping on a fine glass of champagne in Searcys Bar, St Pancras International Station with another member of the sales team, we celebrated the success of a long, arduous week at the company's annual exhibition. *"Cheers!"* Waiting for our train back home we clinked glasses, a well-deserved treat for getting through the past five days. We knew the hard work had only just begun, the following few months would be challenging, as we tried to sell in a targeted number of the following year's ranges to customers.

Travelling alone had never really bothered me, perhaps the nature of my past work had helped me to conquer any fears, but I also found it quite liberating, a time to reflect, mull situations over in my mind. I pulled out a piece of scrap paper from my handbag I had used earlier to make a note of my lodgings for that evening. I don't know where the words came from, but they flowed with ease from my pen, directly underneath the address details of the Hasting's bed and breakfast accommodation. Reading back the poem to myself, I was startled at how effortless the composition had been, my first creative piece of writing and unbeknown to me then, the first seeds of a new journey in my life. From childhood I had always been a keen scribbler, keeping diaries, concocting short silly verses in close family and friend's birthday cards, however, this was something different. Not only did my works of art become more frequent, but I think writing the poetry may have been contributory to my healing too.

Not long after returning back from my short trip, the holiday mode was soon replaced by boredom, then very quickly into despair. As time went by the days grew exceedingly long, the evenings even longer, until the hours of lightness and darkness intertwined with each other in a blurred vision, mashed up by my increasing alcohol consumption. I had always enjoyed a drink, maybe a little more than I should sometimes, however, it tended to be a social pastime, which generally took place at the weekend to celebrate the end of a long, arduous working week. My mental state was deteriorating rapidly, but although depression had played an annoying game with me since my late teens, this time the illness was becoming frighteningly worse and neither the anti-depressants, food binging, or drinking was making me feel better.

During this time though I continued to put pen to paper, sometimes verse, other times a paragraph or two in reference to my thoughts, all of which I eventually transferred onto my lap top into appropriately named files. A portfolio of poetry, blogs, with even the first creative seedlings for a possible book, this book 'There Is a Way' began to build and yet apart from a few Face-Book shares, I never considered this could be my free ticket to a much more meaningful life. Initially the play on words were almost always very dark, but sometimes my bona fide playful nature would creep to the surface allowing some of my compositions to be exceedingly funny too. Constantly writing, painlessly scribbling notes, until this in itself almost became an obsession. For a few months I sat until the early hours of the morning thinking up story lines for a still unfinished fictional novel called 'The Return of Mary Cartwright.' It seemed far easier to transpose some of my dilemmas onto the imaginary character who played the lead role in my narrative, which I am sure many authors do. I was so very messed up, but realise now that this was a crucial release channel for my emotions and feelings during possibly the lowest point in my life.

It was April 28th 2011, just over a year since my redundancy and I was still without a job. I had been offered a number of sales positions, probably due to the track record with my previous company. There was little doubt I could get results, but on the two occasions I accepted fresh challenges from potential future employers, I barely lasted more than a few weeks. My heart was no longer in a career I had fought so hard to achieve for eighteen years, however, time was running out, so I needed to find something and quickly.

My redundancy money pot was almost empty, which had not only been helping me to make ends meet, but was also keeping up my IVA payments to keep the creditors at bay. I hadn't felt it was necessary to tell the finance company my latest predicament, because I was so sure I would find another job before the money ran out. How wrong could I have been. I tested out new waters and in-between these failures, I signed on at the job centre with thousands of others. Nothing seemed to work, behind closed doors I was becoming seriously ill, worrying about the bills, the remaining debt, my home and consequently my life.

"Shit, here we go!" I screwed up my eyes, hardly daring to peep between the gaps reluctantly created with my fingers and with both feet now firmly on the bathroom scales, I watched in horror. The digits shot from zero, passing eight stone, nine stone, and ten stone, resting on eleven stone three. *"Where had my perfect figure gone?"* The dreaded spare tyre, which seems perfectly acceptable to go hand in hand with midlife, began to jiggle and wobble as I stepped down from the scales feeling disgusted with myself. I had been notified once more that I was over two stone heavier than my ideal weight and this didn't make the start to a perfect day. Muttering under my breath, I reminded myself of the hard facts *"You have no life, no*

job, no man, and no children. Very soon you will have no home; therefore, being two stone heavier is the least of your worries."

The mirror tells no lies and this particular spring morning was no exception. I stared long and hard at the image looking back at me begging for answers. With my roots inches thick, eyes swollen from a never- ending lack of sleep, the same question repeated its self over and over again *"Why me?"* I could feel the increasing tension throughout every inch of my body, as I moved closer to inspect my complexion. With my head pounding, I stroked my cheeks, then pulled and stretched the sides of my eyes. I had always been so proud of my youthful skin, but lines were now starting to appear across my face, depicting the story of my folly.

I staggered into the bedroom and flung open the wardrobe door. Although many of the beautiful dresses bought during my spending madness had now been either sold, or given to charity, a few were still hanging from the rail, their sequins, diamantes and glitter now shimmering from the bedroom light. I ran my fingers across a black taffeta ball gown purchased especially for a New Year's Eve trip with friends, but then looked down at my size 12 jeans. Faded and ripped across the knees, I had always felt my best in a pair of denims and now they were almost buried under a pile of leggings and baggy t shirts. I looked back at the handful of remaining designer frocks, a sharp reminder of my past addiction and a reflection of its misconceptions too.

I grabbed a pair of denim look leggings and an old sweatshirt of Dad's, both of which I had worn the previous day. With hardly anything left to fit me, choosing what to wear was a lot less complicated and apart from the odd family get together there was little cause for dressing up anyway. Positioning myself on the edge of the bed I pulled on my leggings, looking towards the door as it creaked open. My cat Maddie peered into the bedroom and meowed as she entered, just to make sure I was aware of her arrival. Her great big saucer eyes stared up at me lovingly as she jumped up beside me, rubbing her head affectionately against my arm. It didn't seem 10 years ago since she had travelled back with me from Liverpool, a six-week old kitten, one of the offspring from an adopted stray cat taken in by my brother's wife. I had fallen in love with the little black and white ball of fluff instantly. Maddie nudged me once more purring loudly, but then snuggled down on my coffee coloured duvet, she appeared to understand that before breakfast I needed to get dressed.

Having pulled on my leggings I gazed longingly at my late Father's sweatshirt. His passing in 2003 had literally brought me to my knees, so retaining and wearing a garment belonging to him seemed to give me some comfort. I missed him terribly, particularly over the past few years and burying my head into the soft black and grey garment, the tears once again tumbled down my cheeks.

"He would have known the answers Maddie, he would have understood, wouldn't he?" Maddie looked up at me sympathetically, watching me weep as she so often did.

Once again I glared at my reflection in the wardrobe mirror, before making my way down the stairs to feed the cat.

"What an absolute mess!"

My hair roots were as overgrown as the garden lawns, my mobile credit almost empty and I knew there wasn't enough money in my bank account to pay all the bills for the following month.

Later that day I made what was possibly a reckless decision, but I couldn't see any other alternative than to cancel all of my direct debits. With the lap top perched on my knees showing a list of payments and due dates from its screen, I hesitated before confirming their deletions one by one. Once I had completed the process, dripping with sweat and overcome by nausea through guilt I nervously logged out of my online banking service. It was still early afternoon, but the only friend I thought I could lean on, my one solace was an unopened bottle of red wine, however, within almost an hour I was pouring the last droplets into my glass as the tears tumbled from my eyes. I just couldn't seem to get throughout a day without crying.

I looked around the house as though it was for the last time. I had nothing left of extreme value, anything with even the tiniest potential of raising funds to help me stay afloat financially was continually being considered for eBay. A Marilyn Monroe picture hung centre stage in the living room and she smiled at me, just as she always did. Her ruby red lips, pale flawless face and beautiful blonde hair, the picture had witnessed so much over the past eleven years since I purchased it from a small collectables shop in Leicestershire. I barely had anything left of the Hollywood star's memorabilia and this would probably be the next to go.

I tipped the empty wine glass into my mouth, hoping to catch the last few dregs that had settled into the bottom. A huge big knot, which for months seemed to have lodged itself firmly in the middle of my chest, suddenly started to rise and form a lump in my throat. It was then my outpouring of sorrow came, but unlike before, these tears were inconsolable, grief stricken and uncontrollable. I screamed and wailed for the next few hours, feeling completely desolate and utterly heartbroken.

"What had gone wrong with my life?"

Contemplating suicide is not something I wish to remind

myself of, but particularly during those latter few months there were a number of occasions when I was alone, numbed by the effects of drink and anti-depressants, I considered it as an option. Even though I fully understood the devastating impact it would have on the family and friends I left behind, I still felt it was the best solution for everyone. Still sobbing I pulled down both the Prozac and painkillers, feeling even more determined that taking my life was the only way. I Studied the packaging and contents for a short while, but then realised I needed more wine to wash them down, so after throwing the pills on the kitchen table I grabbed my purse and waterproof coat.

"This one is very nice and has a special offer this week." I could hear her friendly voice in the distance as she pointed towards a bottle of Shiraz, whilst I loitered nervously around the collection of red wines. It was still early evening and I had walked to one of the three local convenience stores situated near where I lived. Ashamed of what was possibly turning into yet another addiction, I shared my daily visits to each of the shops equally.

"Or perhaps you might like the merlot?" The shop assistant once again interrupted my thoughts. To be perfectly honest, what type of grape hardly mattered to me anymore, but guided by her choices I went with the first option and clutching a carrier bag filled with an assortment of carbohydrate delights and a red Australian Shiraz, I headed back home.

Turning the key of the front door, I breathed a sigh of relief as I stepped inside the house and slammed it shut behind me. I needed to be certain no one ever knew my secret, however, the only visitor I generally received late in the evenings was the pizza boy delivering my order.

I rushed upstairs, changing into the only pyjamas I had left to fit around my ever-increasing waistline. With Maddie close at my heels, the telephone started to ring as I made my way back down the staircase. This was Mum's third call of the day and thankfully I was back from the shop in time to receive it.

"How are you?" "What are you up too?" My annoyance at the questions she asked simply stemmed from shame and as I walked into the kitchen with the receiver against my ear, I once again lied.

"I'm feeling so much better today Mum. Thought I might come and spend the day with you tomorrow."

It was six pm with the silver coloured wall clock. Maddie eager for her tea was meowing by my feet, so making the cat's need for food an excuse to her, we said our good byes.

"I'll call you later Sharon, before getting into bed." Mum's last words rang in my ears as I placed the telephone receiver on the kitchen table and picked up the pill packets once more.

The following day was a Bank Holiday, though that barely held any significance with me anymore. Every day just seemed the same, no matter what the occasion. There was never anything of importance, or consequence derived from one hour to the next. As a member of the British workforce I had always relished Bank Holidays, in particular the late August one. Weather permitting, I would generally meet up with friends during the day and we would enjoy drinks in the late summer sunshine. This all seemed in the long distant past though, as my desire to mix with colleagues other than Marie had waned considerably. Usually a social butterfly, my self-confidence was dropping at a rate of knots, I couldn't seem to handle people in the way I used to, misjudging and always sceptical of their motives.

Up until the end of 2010 I had been involved in organising a few events at a mate's bar, this helped me to mingle and meet new acquaintances. I had also hoped it could be a spring board to a different career, choosing to set up in self-employment under the business name 'Monroe Events.' My past charity events were always successful, but sadly transferring my marketing and coordinating skills into this type of work was never meant to be. 'A Christmas Ball' one of the last function's I was involved with, I did not even attend the occasion, instead I sat at home drinking wine and feeling sorry for myself, whilst I disgracefully allowed my Mum and Marie to stand in my place.

The eve of a special bank holiday, which had been given by the state because Prince William, a possible future King of England was to marry Kate Middleton. No doubt, probably the happiest time of their lives, but for me April 29th 2011 perhaps wouldn't even be another day in my calendar.

I curled up on the huge brown sofa holding a family bag of crisps in one hand and the first glass from my second bottle of wine in the other. Reminiscent of a clip from the 'Bridget Jones' movie, but yet waking up in the small hours of the morning still clutching an empty wine glass was certainly more in line with an AA advertisement, warning of the symptoms to look out for. The times I had been aroused from an alcohol-induced sleep, both startled and scared from either the telephone, or Maddie's gentle tapping against my leg. The sound of Mum's voice frantic to know if there was a problem, because she had called me a number of times without any answer, or Maddie's big eyes staring up at me, wondering why I had missed bedtime. Sometimes if I managed to stagger up the stairs, I would find her curled up on my side of the bed, snoring softly. Maddie had obviously given up and retired without me.

I poured my second glass of wine and looking over at the pill packets laying by my side as I contemplated the next day. The country's jubilations and celebrations would be in full flow, but did I really care? I wanted so badly to find some sort of peace, a way out of the turmoil, however, solutions seemed very thin on the ground.

There have been a few times in my life where all things felt incomprehensible, high above these though was admitting to myself Mum's increasing awareness to my suffering. I picked up the pill packets and clutched them tightly to my chest. I knew I needed to end this quickly, or tell her the truth. Mum's heart was breaking and losing my home could not be any closer to reality, so it was time to accept defeat, whichever way I chose to do it.

CHAPTER 10
SINGLE BED

'She lost her home, she lost all she had
And what to do she couldn't be sure,
But from the bottom there is only up
And this is where her life did restore.'

I didn't take my life that night, because once more the alcohol got the better of me. Instead I woke up in the early hours of the morning still upright, sat on the sofa with my head almost buried in my chest, clutching the pill packets tightly in my hand. My body seemed to sway from side to side as I staggered clumsily to my feet, kicking over the wine glass I had precariously left by my side. The residual Shiraz seeped across the wooden floor and I stared for a few seconds watching the stream of red wine heading towards the living room carpet. Feeling disgusted with myself, I picked up the empty glass and stumbled into the kitchen. Placing both the glass and the tablets onto the dining table, I glanced over at the clock, which was now showing the time to be 4.30am.

My suicide plot had once again failed, but maybe the intention to take my life was never strong enough. I am sure there has always been a spark of wisdom within me, even though perhaps through lack of use I may have reduced it to a mere flicker, but how long had this logic been desperately fighting to push through all my madness. I knew my conscience could no longer deal with all the deceit and this was why I continued to give my GP umpteen excuses to prolong my prescription of anti-depressants. It was also the reason I was drinking to excess. I almost wanted to block out the quieter, gentler voice of reason inside my head, telling me there is a way and yet I seemed to delight in listening to the less comforting, harsher voices yelling at me there was nothing I could do, my situation would never change and that no one was interested in my predicament anyway. It was tough enough to acknowledge how reliant I had become on alcohol, but even more distressing for me to accept the reasons why I constantly felt the need to be intoxicated.

Remembering the wine spillage, I walked unsteadily over to the cleaning cupboard and pulled out a cloth to wipe clean the living room's blood red stained floor. The trail of Shiraz seemed to have just stopped short of the brown and cream carpet, which was quite a relief, so after mopping up the knocked over wine I threw the soiled cloth into the kitchen sink and clambered up the stairs to bed. It hardly seemed worth laying my head on the pillow with almost less than an hour before sunrise. I could hear the birds singing and the dawn light was already starting to creep through a crack in the bedroom curtains, however, if I was finally going to face Mum later that day, I knew I would need a clear head.

It was hard to say how long Maddie had been fast asleep on the bed. Curled up with her head resting on the far side pillow, she didn't take too kindly to the disturbance, but after finally ending my struggle with the duvet cover, I managed to sneak into the bed by her side. The weight of her black and white furry body on top of the quilt had made it an exceedingly strenuous task, nevertheless, she didn't see it that way and looked up at me in utter disgust.

I have grown up surrounded by family pets and in particular cats. It is true what they say about the feline species though, they do have a tendency to think what's yours is theirs and my cat more than exemplified this idea. Maddie believed she had rights to every corner of the house, all three bedrooms and if she could beat me to it, my side of the bed. Spoilt, adored and totally loved, she nearly always got away with it too.

It was almost ten o clock when the distant sound of ringing disturbed my sleep and as I began to stir I immediately recognized the shrill repetitive tone to be my bedside telephone. I clambered for the receiver, noticing Maddie was no longer sharing the bed. She had probably tried to awaken me shortly after I crept in beside her, but obviously the few gentle taps on my forehead with her paw had not been successful, so she must have retired downstairs in a sulk. From a kitten Maddie had grown accustomed to my early morning starts, unfortunately though, although 5.30am alarm calls had long been unnecessary in my world, in her world past habits seemed hard to relinquish.

Mum was already on the other end of the line asking if I was coming to see her, as I had promised the day before. She seemed quite concerned I was still in bed, but somehow I managed to convince her I had been writing long into the early hours of the morning. More lies, more fabricated stories to cover up my descent into a self-destructing life style, a way of living that eventually could only end in disaster. Cringing, I put down the receiver after confirming to Mum I would be with her in the next couple of hours.

The butterflies were already starting to gather in my stomach, because I knew it was time to come clean. I couldn't continue in this way any longer. Already completely drained of everything, lacking in energy and without any future resources for income, I was fast running out of options. There seemed nothing worthwhile to cling onto anymore, as I realised all my hopes and dreams had been wiped from under my feet, the social position I had strived for stripped away from me through my own sheer stupidity, but did all the blame just lie with me. What about the banks, the financial system, which had encouraged me to pump up my loans, max out my credit cards without too many questions about my ability to repay? Sometimes it had taken one short phone call and within an hour a credit limit was increased.

I do hold my hands up to my lack of responsibility during those thirty years, however, the assumption we can never rebuild and that most situations are totally out of our control is a fallacy which needs to be addressed. We have the power to deal with many circumstances effectively, but even external events we are not able to influence can still be handled more positively by changing the way we feel about ourselves. If we have more faith in our own capabilities, this then shifts our perception, so that we are less likely to judge other people unfairly, or write off difficult conditions, automatically regarding any solutions to the problem as hopeless. We are also able to assess incidents in a much broader context, making our role in life far easier to understand.

The only time we stop loving is when we lose faith in ourselves.'

Okay, so I hadn't found the love of my life, I didn't have children, I hadn't got a job and I was also up to my eyes in debt, but it was totally absurd to believe my situation to be any more burdensome than anyone else's sorrow and how completely defeatist to think my troubles were totally irreversible. Apart from a misguided analysis of my predicament, often exaggerated by the regular intake of alcohol and prescribed pills, my gifted qualities were far from inadequate. These personal experiences were real, but I needed to gain strength from them instead of wallowing in self-pity. If I was ever going to lift myself from out of the present setup, it was also necessary for me to step outside of the box, develop new skills and enhance the talents I had already been blessed with. It was time for reflection and to remember it had always been sheer determination, which got me through every obstruction whenever my back was up against a wall. Since leaving school I had proved time and time again that even without qualifications, or any initial ambition, a life can be transformed. If I was interested enough about a goal, or a challenge nothing would hold me back. I would passionately read, study and practice, soaking up every piece of information like a sponge.

> *'I may not have an O Level*
> *An A Level or Degree,*
> *I may not be a Doctor*
> *High class or bourgeoisie,*
> *But one thing that I know for sure*
> *There's one thing I understand,*
> *That life is how you make it*
> *How you take the stuff unplanned.'*

Telling Mum about my financial predicament is probably the hardest decision I have ever had to make, however, she was surprisingly very understanding about my situation, but Mum also delivered what must have been the most difficult revelation about her and Dad. A secret they had kept hidden for many years, one that made it so much clearer why she could show me such deep compassion and sympathy for what I was going through.

"This is grim Sharon, but we will deal with this together now. You are no longer on your own!"

Hearing about Dad's bankruptcy was devastating. It was a few months after the birth of my younger sibling brother Paul and the consequences for the both of them were horrendous. Dad had worked in the painting and decorating trade from school, so after achieving his City and Guilds he decided to set up his own company. Due to a number of outstanding payments and theft from some of his workforce, the business sadly collapsed leaving my parents riddled in debt.

There may have been some naivety on Dad's part, he was young and wanted to make his way in life, but like any entrepreneur with a family to look after, his heart was in the right place. My parents need not have gone through what they did, surely my Father could have been helped, guided through his company's financial catastrophe, but instead all he and his wife could look forward to was fear, heartache and so much humiliation. Mum chokingly told me that she would hide under the table when the knocks came on the door from the bailiffs. Quaking at the memory, she also bravely called to mind how after the creditors had cruelly taken away all their household goods to pay off some of the outstanding debts, she was then given the first option to buy back some of their unsold furniture.

"They could not charge me a lot" she recalled *"because we hadn't got the money."*

Understandably these recollections were difficult for her, but in trying to console me she relived every dreadful moment.

I have no doubt the stress of the bankruptcy is what probably triggered the numerous illnesses which plagued my Dad's life and I was once again convinced after hearing Mum's terrifying confession that the society we grow up in is never too keen to help out in our times of failure, but will almost always be extremely quick to embrace our feelings of inadequacy, if we allow it to. It made me think back to my own experiences, when I had to tolerate a number of immensely cold hearted and very often callous telephone callers from the bank's debt collecting agencies. Without fully understanding my situation, a few of their staff gave the impression through their interrogative nature of delighting in my misery. Their faceless harsh voices on the other end of the line, seeming to enjoy their conjured up feelings of superiority, with their only intention to kick me down further by answering me in a cruel and cutting manner when I explained I had no money to pay off the debt. I certainly could associate with what my parents must have gone through, but all those years ago the animosity must have been so much greater. These types of uncomfortable incidences certainly leave their mark on many unsuspecting victims, which is why we tend to be so much more critical of ourselves when things go wrong in our lives.

Mum understood I wanted to keep my independence, so initially she tried to help me by subsidizing my bills and rent payments, however, this was never going to work on a permanent basis without some form of income. I was still not in the best shape, but with no idea what I wanted to do with the rest of my life, finding and maintaining a job was proofing extremely difficult.

During this time, I continued to write, publishing my verse on social media under the guise of 'Pisces Lady', even composing and selling some bespoke poetry for weddings and christenings. The creations I made to make money I found the most laborious to produce, but I think this is because it hadn't come from the heart. I needed to earn a living though, so the small amounts I made from this type of verse contributed a little towards the household bills.

I eventually set up my own website, however, this didn't seem to change the negative outcome from my countless submissions to agents, publishers and magazines. Hundreds of rejections and yet family and friends seemed to love my work, but it wasn't just family and friends I needed to impress. If I was to be taken seriously by anyone in the literacy world, then my work had to reach a much wider audience and this was a hurdle which was necessary for me to jump over. Having also registered the truthful reality that poetry alone wasn't going to get my name on the high street's book shelves, I decided to submit the first three chapters of my fictional story 'The Return of Mary Cartwright.' Once again though the returned emails only contained polite refusals and I started to draw a blank as to where my creativity was heading, if it was going anywhere at all. I nonchalantly carried on writing though, it was as if I knew that one day everything I had gone through, all the knock backs, brick walls and rejections would eventually make sense.

In the meantime, although in myself I was slowly getting much stronger, my financial dilemma was becoming increasingly worse, so towards the end of 2011 I put the small amount of furniture I had left into storage, packed my bags and reluctantly waved goodbye to my independence. I had no choice, it was the only thing I could do. With a doting Mother to take me under her wing, I considered myself extremely lucky, as I realised without her help I could have been dead, or at least homeless and on the streets. Mum even offered to let me have her double bedroom whilst she took residence in the visitor's box bedroom, but I was adamant she had already done more than enough, so it was back to a single bed occupancy for me.

We celebrated the New Year in her small two bedroomed bungalow vowing 2012 would be a turning point in my life, because we were able to face the issues together. Before Christmas I had finally contacted the IVA company, explaining I was no longer able to continue with my payments. The agent was extremely considerate to my change of circumstances and over the next few months' meetings were arranged with my creditors to see if they would accept what I had already paid as a final payment, writing off the rest. All but one agreed, which infuriatingly turned it into a failed IVA plan, cancelling out everything I had already paid. I would once again be vulnerable to my creditors if I didn't seek help, so once the festivities were over Mum came with me to the Citizens Advice to find out what could be done. A small payment plan was put in place and the rebuilding of my life had begun, but I don't think I could have ever anticipated the transformations that were about to take place over the next couple of years.

CHAPTER 11
EXCHANGE OF APPLES

*'Her values seem to have changed somewhat
Which initially scared her half to death,
See she always thought she knew herself
But now with time to take a breath...'*

Over the new year I had been completely enveloped in a recently purchased book, which seemed to explain true happiness perfectly, however, also taking the time to digest numerous articles about humanity's misconception and obsession with success, I could see where I had been going horribly wrong. Written by a British author, it soon became apparent to me that the writer ran various workshops and one that instantly struck a chord with me was her meditation course. Having already tried to master the concept, I wasn't over confident that I was meditating correctly, so thinking I may need some expert guidance I decided to book myself onto the Sunday morning Workshop. Mum kindly offered to pay for my expenses, she knew I was really intrigued by the practise and thought it could only be of help with my recovery. Having heard me rave about the positive results it can have in changing years of negative thinking, she wholeheartedly encouraged me to consider meditation as a further option to enhance my well-being.

I had already been taking enthusiastic steps to regain control of my life by slowly weaning myself from the dependency of anti-depressants and confining my drinking to nights out with friends, or family get-togethers. But it was during a night out with friends, after months shunning social events, I discovered my partying days were also well and truly over. It had been a wonderful evening sampling the various wine bars and bistros in one of Sheffield's more fashionable areas, however, finding it difficult to keep up with the pace, I later embarrassingly fell asleep in a night club whilst the rest of my colleagues danced into the early hours. This was when I realised my likes, dislikes and perceptions were starting to change dramatically. My metamorphosis was beginning to take place, transforming the person that I had long grown accustomed to, into someone else. A total stranger even to me and I am not sure if I was yet fully ready for such a significant shift in lifestyle.

'She barely knew herself at all
But behind the wit, the style and charm,
She was hiding her authentic self
Her vulnerability kept safe from harm!'

It was a beautiful Spring Sunday morning in May 2012 as I began my journey from South Kensington into Chelsea. Although it seemed a fair walking distance to where the meditation class was being held, I knew I had plenty of time, so I wanted to capitalize on the warm sunshine and the auspicious sights of London town.

Halfway to my destination and I decided to stop off at a charming little bistro to quench my thirst. Enjoying the sunshine on my face I lazily watched the fresh lemon slices and ice cubes gently bobbing around the top of my glass. I had been served by the cutest waiter, who had not only delivered me the cool sparkling water, but had made my day even more perfect by showering me with a multitude of lovely compliments too.

I graciously accepted his praise and taking a sip from the ice cold drink, my mind, driven by the young waiter's recent flattery proceeded to wander down memory lane. Remembering my first holiday abroad with friends, away from the watchful eye of our parents, I recaptured our frivolity, being almost sent giddy by the charming words dished out from the local boys. Fresh faced eighteen-year-olds enticed by romantic gestures from the young men of Tenerife, eager to bed yet more gullible English roses. Needless to say my first holiday romance with a somewhat dubious Spanish waiter was not at all momentous, but I did pick up a few educational tips, learning the hard way that some young men are not to be trusted.

We are all guilty from a lack of judgement sometimes, we are all prone to making irresponsible decisions too, especially in our younger years. Immaturity clouds our vision, because we think we know it all and yet we understand so little. If we study hard enough at school we leave with a number of qualifications, however, is this enough to steer a future generation along the right course. I don't think it is, but if the educational system's targets have been achieved, a good job seems to have been done for the youth of our society.

Mistakes are part and parcel of growing up, a prerequisite of life and although some of our errors we can perhaps look back on without any cause for concern, sadly from my own experiences this is not always the case. We must be able to smile at our blunders, interpret the message they have delivered, digest and capitalise from the knowledge in their lesson, because this will then enable us to move through every stage of our existence with very little to fear. I was confident meditation could help me do this, but feel even more convinced that it should be included in every child's school curriculum after reaping sensational health benefits in both body and mind from just over three years of practise. However, once again triggered by my own occurrences, I also hold another belief that nothing is ever too late to bring into our lives, especially if it encourages peace of mind, compassion and kindness.

'Nothing is too late; the time is always right for positive change.'

Something seemed very special about that Sunday in May 2012, a sense of calmness and tranquillity radiated around me, therefore even the lengthy wait for my change and receipt from the payment of the sparking water, didn't seem to alter my mood. The waiter finally returned full of apologies for his drawn out absence, suggesting cheekily he was trying to prolong my stay at the bistro.

Having checked out the whereabouts of the venue earlier, I knew I hadn't far to go and my excitement began to take hold. Somehow I knew this was going to be the most amazing experience for me. I felt sure after this introductory course I would adopt the practice of meditation, so that it would become a part of my daily routine to benefit my health, rather than my past destructive habits that threatened to endanger it. I had registered that as a person, I was changing, already becoming observant to the many things that no longer impressed me, which I once classed as ultra-important.

A perfect example was my unusually brisk walk through Harrods the previous day. It had been impossible for me to catch a train early enough on the Sunday morning to make the workshop on time, so after settling into my hotel room I decided to make the most of a late Saturday afternoon. Choosing to take a leisurely stroll into Knightsbridge, I stalled as I approached the store's grand entrance. For old time's sake I nervously passed by the shop's welcoming doorman and stepped into the stylish accessories department, where I soon realised the excitable adrenalin rush that used to wash over me, had been replaced by a nonchalant, laid back attitude. The smell of expensive perfume, designer handbags perfectly displayed with fancy evening gloves and diamante necklaces to encourage multiple purchases, barely caused me to raise my eyebrows. It had been extremely tough to overcome the powerful, impulsive urges which had me continually reaching for my credit cards, but to discover I could no longer be influenced by the alluring atmosphere, glamour and assistants dressed from head to toe in the latest fashion trends was such a relief. None of this had anything to do with my inability to spend on plastic and neither was I frustrated by my financial constraints, my desire to buy these types of luxuries had simply vanished. I could not even be tempted to peruse the quality goods, let alone purchase any of them. This was just one aspect of my life that was turning itself on its head and as I watched my dreams turn upside down, I often had to pinch myself to check I was still Sharon Bull.

After the meditation workshop, I walked casually back towards South Kensington Tube Station with a colleague I had met on the course. We bid our goodbyes at the entrance of the underground and he disappeared into the bustling crowd, whilst I continued the rest of my journey to the hotel. I felt wonderfully strange, a feeling hard to explain as I sauntered along the streets of London, soaking up the mid afternoon sunshine with a flower gripped tightly in one hand and a fresh juicy green apple tucked safely in my small cloth handbag. Both had been offered to me as gifts at the meditation class to symbolise abundance and happiness.

I had planned to stay another evening having arranged to meet someone special for tea. I couldn't have possibly called it a romance, although he generally told me what I wanted to hear and I suppose for quite some time this had been comforting for my bruised and battered ego. Our relationship had developed in the midst of my turmoil and we initially connected whilst I was also eagerly searching

'Myspace' for musicians to get involved with my latest charity show. Our direct messaging over the internet, particularly in the early hours of the morning soon became more frequent and as his status claimed he was single, I had no reason to doubt any other. I have to remember our friendship began during 2010 when I was down on my heels, feeling the lowest of the low, gullible and desperately in need of someone to show me love. Someone, who I felt understood me, yet had no idea about the tragedy that was going on in my life. Not really the basis for a true meaningful relationship, but it gave me a few specks of hope, which seemed to lighten my mood a little.

I glanced at my mobile to check if I had received a return text from my teatime date. Nothing, but that wasn't unusual and neither was the sight of a homeless person huddled in a doorway either, particularly in London. As I passed by the lady, who looked to be middle aged our lives seemed to connect together. For a few seconds it was as though we were fused into one being, almost as if I had been allowed to touch her soul, so I could appreciate her journey, the way she was being forced to exist.

I stopped in my tracks stifled by an overwhelming urge to show her some kindness and with tears in my eyes I turned around to approach the homeless lady. It was then I sadly realised how little she had, as I watched her tightly cling onto what seemed to be her only possession, a tired looking ruck sack that probably doubled up as a pillow to rest her head when darkness fell.

"Would you like an apple?" I asked her.

I quickly pulled the fresh juicy green apple from my bag and handed it over to her. I have never seen such gratitude in someone's eyes as she thanked me. I walked away with tears falling down my cheeks whilst she eagerly tucked into the fruit.

Once back in my room I couldn't seem to get the middle aged homeless lady out of my mind, however, I had an idea, but first I needed to pop my flower into a glass of water. I checked my mobile phone once more for any messages, then headed back out towards a supermarket I had spotted close by the hotel. Once inside the store I moved swiftly up and down the aisles filling up a handbasket with various foods and drink. Sandwiches, crisps, water, orange juice, cake and fruit, the lady in the doorway deserved to have a tea-time meal just as much as I did. Thankfully, she was still there when I returned to her spot with the two carrier bags of goodies, although initially, I don't think she could quite believe her eyes. It didn't take her too long to grasp she wasn't dreaming though, so it was heart-warming to leave her smiling, enthusiastically unpeeling one of the sandwich wrappers.

Back at the hotel, it came as no surprise when I finally received a message of apology, with numerous excuses why my date couldn't make it for tea, but I wasn't going to let the disappointment ruin what had so far been a beautiful day. Besides, I was in an unusually relaxed frame of mind, which I feel sure had been brought about through a combination of walking, sunshine and meditation, therefore after eating a wholesome meal complimented by a gorgeously tasting glass of red wine, I was more than ready to hit the sheets.

The following morning, I meditated alone for the first time in my hotel room on the 27th floor. I set my mobile timer for twenty minutes, then closed my eyes after looking out at the most awesome view of the capital city. To clear my mind, I began repeating the mantra I was given at the workshop, which opened floodgates that were generally locked, bolted and screwed down, allowing calmness and tranquillity to wash over every inch of my being. A strange experience, but yet I sensed if I incorporated the practise into my daily life, eventually it would help me to analyse past, present and future events much more clearly, allowing the remainder of my journey to be a far happier and fulfilling experience.

Packed and ready for my journey home, I glanced around the bedroom one more time to check if I had left anything behind. The gorgeous flower I had been given at the workshop was blossoming in the glass of water, so I didn't have the heart to stunt its growth by packing into my case. Instead I left it on the dressing table top with a note for the cleaner saying *'Please look after this flower, enjoy its beauty!'* Neither of the gifts given to me on the course did I take home with me, not the fresh juicy green apple, or the flower.

I stood by the lift waiting to be taken from the dizzy heights of the hotel's top floor, down to their ground floor reception. In my white denim jacket with matching cut-off jeans, I looked over at the black and white Mary Quant style luggage by my side and smiled. Contrast had always been of the essence to me, down to every last minor detail, so even my suitcases needed to compliment the outfit I was wearing.

I almost missed one of the hotel staff as he breezed past me, cheerily bidding me good morning, but what happened immediately after this was more than strange. He suddenly stopped in his tracks, turned back around and came towards me holding a huge bowl in his hands, brimming with fresh juicy green apples.

'Would you like an apple Madam?' I could barely hear the words.

An extraordinary and surreal moment for me, however, with my mouth still wide open in shock, I gratefully pulled out a fresh juicy green apple from the top of the pile. I thanked the young man, tucked it safely into my small cloth handbag, whilst at the same time trying hard to convince myself that the incident had actually just happened.

Could this have been what is called 'The Law of Attraction', which I had read so much about, or was it purely coincidence that at the same time I had been waiting for a lift on the 27th floor of the hotel, a member of staff walked by with a bowl of fresh juicy green apples. Not a bowl of bananas, or even red apples, but a bowl of fresh juicy green apples. My feelings in regards to the homeless lady in the doorway had been so powerful, so it was a little bit scary to think that the hotel worker had almost mirrored my actions from the day before. Neither a sceptic, nor a believer of 'The Law of Attraction', what I did decide after the incident was to keep an open mind and educate myself even more.

It is our choice what we choose to believe, nothing has any power over our mind, unless we choose to let our many unsubstantiated perceptions take control. I had allowed this to happen far too often, always presuming the worst case scenario, regularly jumping to the wrong conclusions assuming my value, or point of view was of little consequence.

This was where I had hoped the meditation would help me gain some strength, but after a number of months religiously bringing the discipline into my daily activity, I became extremely worried. There seemed to be a sudden increase in my frustrations, my self-loathing peaked, rather than diminished and my anger outbursts were becoming much more frequent. I could not understand why this was happening, however, after speaking to a number of learned people two important issues came to light. Firstly, from the meditation practises my awareness was becoming more astute, therefore I was becoming an observer to my thoughts and the way they made me feel emotionally, which would answer why I was conscious of my frustrations, self-loathing and anger outbursts.

Secondly, to explain what was happening to me, my mind was simulated to a small pond, which because it had been left dormant for many years, the mud and whatever else had settled at the bottom had long been undisturbed and well hidden. The meditation process was likened to a big wooden stick stirring the pond, unsettling everything at the bottom, therefore bringing it to the surface. In other words, my years of mindless thinking, hidden fears and buried grievances were now all staring me in the face, so that I could deal with them head on.

Meditation has become a huge part of my life and I will never give up the practise knowing how it has helped to change my life. I weathered the storm as suggested to me, holding onto the theory that sometimes things have to get worse, before they get better. We live in a world which seems to expect too much, too soon and patience doesn't seem to be tolerated enough. We seem to give up our dreams so easily, lose heart if we fall at the first hurdle and yet success if we are extremely lucky is generally derived from months of hard work, but more often than not years of trial and error.

The romance never fully blossomed with my cancelled tea time date, but then when relationships are not meant to be, especially if they become embroiled in lies and deceit the best option is to walk away. Unfortunately, I didn't close the door soon enough and anger can so easily creep into the equation, especially when you have just stirred a small pond that has been dormant for many years through meditation. I became extremely bitter in the way our friendship was handled towards the end, however, for me there is no longer any blame.

If only we had the strength in difficult times to embrace patience, take a few deep breaths and simply count to ten before we respond, how different would some of our scenario's possibly end.

CHAPTER 12
TURNING POINT

"So the Prozac went back to the pharmacy,
She didn't need it because she was calm you see,
And creativity became her best chum,
Whilst negativity she kicked up the bum!"

Mum and I started to rebuild my life together. I had gained so much wisdom from the past few years, but a couple of key issues needed to be properly addressed if I was going to finally turn the corner. Throughout my career, no matter what I achieved, or how far up the ladder I climbed, I never once felt the same sense of purpose that I did when I was organizing and planning my charity events. Surely my passionate commitment to worthy causes should have been an indication of where my heart and soul was best suited, however, like many more, my working life was spent mindlessly in the fast lane, so it would never have dawned on me to contemplate, or consider a change in direction.

During the latter few years I had also found that being creative gave me a new kind of energy, a stimulation which was not only beneficial for my mind, but for my well being too. Once again this couldn't have been a clearer message that I needed to use my writing talents to make my way in the world and even more poignantly, my blogs and verse had taken up a new format, sending out messages of hope to others, whilst also raising awareness about issues close to my heart. There had to be a way of incorporating what I loved into what I did for a living, however, with not much idea of how to channel all this new found knowledge, I still needed to earn some money.

I signed on with a temping agency in order to get some

work and it wasn't long before I received my first engagement. Two weeks' holiday relief, managing a switch board with a few various other administration tasks, probably a lot less responsibility than I had been previously used too, but it didn't matter to me, I no longer wanted the worry, or burden attached to more powerful roles. Besides I was writing so much more and this type of job would not overshadow what I loved doing the most.

Unfortunately, my receptionist role didn't last very long as on my second assignment I walked out of the business after being severely and publically scolded by the manager. She had reason to be cross, admittedly I had missed a couple of emails whilst busy writing, one in particular which she seemed to believe was extremely important, but the public humiliation from the mishandled reprimand I couldn't accept. A stark reminder of how corporate hierarchy can often inflate a person's ego, giving them a deluded sense of superiority to excuse ill-judged actions towards their staff. To be honest I had encountered much worse, so maybe I could have battled it out, stood my ground and completed the appointment, but my heart wasn't in it anyway. I knew I wasn't making things easy for myself by walking out and the chances of more recruitment from the temping agency would be slim, but did I really want more of this type of work; I don't think I did. Needless to say my time at the temping agency was brought to an untimely end, as they obviously released me from their books because of the incident.

I cringe when I look back on my working role in sales, thinking about a number of the employer's decisions where I was forced under pressure to accept the situation, even though my disagreement was probably valid. The only solution to me, the only resolution that seemed to make perfect sense was for me to become my own boss, because I doubted I could ever fit into that type of working environment again. Self-employment was not easy though, I had already been made fully aware of this through my abolished events planning business 'Monroe Events.' A small taster of how hellish it is to survive, but as the business folded almost as soon as it had been resurrected, an indicter of how easy it is to give up too.

Since my redundancy in 2010 I had no other option but to claim job seekers allowance on a number of occasions. I hated receiving government handouts with a passion, it wasn't something I had ever been used to. Whenever I walked into the building to sign on at my designated time slot I felt degraded, humiliated about my jobless position and yet there were so many people just like me, all age groups, both sexes from different nationalities feeling the same sense of shame that I was.

Most of the staff were reasonably considerate to people's naturally low self-esteem though, but there had to be one bad apple and unfortunately for me she conducted my first appointment of 2013. For the first time ever I had not fully completed the previous meeting's arranged job finding objectives. It was Christmas time and most of the holidays had been spent with family, but this didn't seem to register has an excuse with the member of staff. She consequently declined my following payment. It was almost as if she had enjoyed depriving a week's pocket money from a naughty school child, using it as a deterrent for future misbehaviour. I was mortified by her smug, cold attitude, but couldn't help thinking how intimidating she would seem with the younger generation. Another kick in the direction towards self-employment, so after writing a letter of complaint to the job centre about the horrid experience, I quit jobseeker payments to venture into what was completely unknown territory to me.

Stepping entirely out of my comfort zone, I almost blagged my way into the motivational speaking circuit, which was a reminder of how I acquired my first sales position. Asked in my interview if I was a competent motorway driver, I immediately responded with what must have been a very convincing affirmative, even though I knew full well I had no experience whatsoever. It worked, because I got the job and inevitably spent the month preceding my start date driving along the various UK motorways with Dad by my side for support.

'Don't let anyone say you can't, because you can,
Ignore what people say and make your plan,
Nothing is impossible
Don't falter, be unstoppable,
Don't let anyone say you can't, because you can!'

Over the next few months I attended numerous networking meetings in order to make some new contacts, whilst at the same time it enabled me to get a feel for the new journey I was about to embark on. There seemed to be quite a few local motivational speakers and coaches, so I tried to get to see as many of them perform as I could, a few held their own workshops and others could be seen doing the circuit of Mind, Body, Spirit shows. I managed to book myself onto a couple of events as a speaker having no idea how I was going to deliver my talk, or even worse what I was going to say. I also organised a couple of events, which was the relatively easy part because of course I had the background knowledge from my previous successful charity events.

However, it was the summer of 2013 when through my involvement with a community radio station I met Paul, who was not only one of the directors of the station, but also a mentor for new business start-ups. Once again I had fearlessly stepped outside the box, when I offered to produce and host a couple of two-hour radio shows during a month's FM window opportunity the station had been given. With limited knowledge, I grasped as much information as I could from a few of the established broadcasters, somehow managing to pull it off. I invited guests to the show, played the music I liked, made a few faux pas, but all in all I actually enjoyed the whole experience having once overcome the fear of the studio's technology. Certain events come into our lives for a reason and although at the time I probably saw myself as the next Jo Whiley, or Vanessa Feltz, it actually sowed the seeds to the next step in my career.

I had so many visions of what my business would look like, but wasn't sure how viable they all were, nevertheless I approached Paul and asked if I could see him, half expecting to come away from the appointment disappointed. Armed with a portfolio containing samples of my written work, business goals and ideas, I don't think I could have been more wrong, he was surprisingly supportive and like me believed I had a concept that could work. I had already written some spoken verse, one in particular, which depicted my life story telling about the depression, addiction, debt and ultimately my ongoing recovery too. I wasn't sure how difficult I would find it, as my knowledge of power point presentations was limited, but I felt almost certain that if I was to combine my verse with images, this would make a far more interesting and innovative talk.

So, in September 2013 having had the privilege of Paul's help and expertise, I officially set up my own business working under the name S.M. Toni. The name had been thought of by my Mum and quite simply represented a combination of close family names. A new website was created through a small local design company, Social Media pages created, talks booked and my minimal power point skills had now been refreshed and refined as I successfully created my first presentation.

After a long discussion with Mum, we both decided it probably wouldn't do me any harm to go public with my story. I was already holding talks and discussing it openly at the events, but this would reach out to a much wider audience, therefore hopefully helping many more to overcome their own personal hurdles. I set about writing a blog detailing my life experiences, before submitting to countless magazines, press agencies and journalists. Patience is always a virtue and I don't think we practice it nearly enough, but this was where I truly and honestly learned never to give up at the first hurdle.

Learning to live on an exceptionally low budget whilst passionately building the foundations of a small business tested my past weaknesses, however I also soon discovered once more that self-employment was by no means an easy ride. This time though I felt so much more determined overcoming and bouncing back from every single knock back, obstacle and rejection.

Whilst all this was going I also grasped what was really important to me, even reigniting some of my childhood passions. From the age of eleven I used to love walking in nature, heading off into the Derbyshire countryside most weekends with my younger brother and a picnic basket. Somehow these kind of simple pleasures disappeared as I grew older, however, with a country park on my doorstep there could never be a better time to bring back into my life, forgotten, yet loved pastimes.

Since twenty I had always been a keen fitness fanatic, yet although I subscribed to all the best gyms I never felt comfortable, they always seemed far too pretentious for me, preferring to train with the guidance of keep fit videos in the privacy of my own home. I loved dancing too and would quite often enjoy my own personal disco, gyrating, spinning and twirling for hours to all my favourite sounds, which surely must have burnt a few hundred calories. Sport on the other hand for me was purely made for watching. I hated participating in any competitive game and would do almost anything at school to get out of playing hockey, or netball. I just wasn't good enough, I even had to play tennis against a wall, because no one selected me for their knock out teams.

Once again though walking and exercise became firmly fixed into my daily routine and alongside meditation all played their part in aiding my recovery. From 2012 the transformation that started to take place both in my thought process and well-being was nothing more than miraculous. But above all this I was finally acknowledging the importance of the creative gift I had been given, cherishing, nurturing and giving my writing the value and worth it deserved by developing a living around it.

I have rarely asked favours from anyone hoping it will get me a few steps higher on the social, or business ladder, because I have always had a strong belief that to feel the benefits of any achievements the hard work has to be put in by ourselves. The only exception to the rule was my charity events, where I would get on my hands and knees for donations and sponsorship. I will always seek advice from sources more learned than myself in a field of interest though, which is exactly what I did when I spoke to a dear and old friend Jools Holland (musician and TV presenter.) He put me in touch with a national poet, who spent a considerable amount of time chatting with me about the literacy world, tips in survival and the pitfalls to watch out for, advice which I not only gratefully appreciated, but also used to further strengthen S.M.Toni's business model.

During my first half century I have known numerous people, who maybe could have lifted me into higher circles, perhaps would have also helped dig me out of the hell hole I fell in too with my addiction, debt and depression, but to me even during shallow times I only ever labelled people that came into my life with one tag *'friend'*, no matter how high, or how low they may have been categorised within society. Not to be used for their importance and neither disregarded for perhaps their lack of ability to do anything for me. We have to remember that no one is better than anyone else, we are each unique, with different talents to share and yet everyone has the same wish, we all want to be happy.

'If we can cherish others over and above ourselves and see their lives as equally important as ours, the world would be a much better place to live in.'

Towards the end of 2013 I finally received a response to one of the innumerable emails I had sent out to various magazines, press agencies and journalists. Not only were they intrigued by my story, but also impressed with how well the detail had been written. The agency concerned was almost certain my experiences, specifically the shopping addiction had all the essential ingredients to interest the national media and so within a few weeks a deal was struck with a national woman's weekly magazine.

In March 2014 my story featured in the Woman's Own magazine, which for many reading what I had gone through in print was a complete shock, but to a few it certainly didn't come as much of a surprise. I covered my tracks well during those dreadful years, in particular the latter few and there was no denying I could put on an elaborate show. Giving out good vibes to those who I felt needed some cheer, a listening ear to others who wanted to offload their anger, or frustrations and a shoulder to cry on for anyone wanting some consolation. Taking the same stance as my dear belated Father, believing wholeheartedly in the words he used to say so often.

"There is always someone worse off than you"

The physical symptoms for someone suffering mental illness can be profound, but unlike a deep wound or a broken leg there is nothing visible for anyone else to see and this makes it easy for a victim of this terrible disease to give the impression they are absolutely fine. However, it is behind closed doors when the affliction tends to kick in, when no one is looking. It is the continual inner suffering, anxiety and torment, which is why it is hard to believe when we hear of celebrities, who seem to have everything are battling with the illness. This is how depression played me, so I feel able to understand why it isn't always detected by others, sometimes until it is too late and why it is still an extremely misunderstood disease.

My story started to gain huge amounts of interest, not only from mental health charities and national well-being movements, but from various radio stations wishing to interview me around Derbyshire, Yorkshire and East Midlands too. I was also finally accepted as a blogger for Huffington Post, after many refused submissions over a period of eighteen months. Another reason to remember never to give up and always have hope.

Maybe the curiosity was because my experiences helped to lift the lid on the toxic effects our society can have on people's lives, whilst at the same time highlighting the huge pressure we put on ourselves as we tirelessly strive to live out the perfect lifestyles seen in magazines, adverts and media. More importantly I also think it was helping to break down the stigma attached to mental illness and how our perceptions of others can be far from their reality.

It was a late sunny afternoon in October 2014 when I skipped out of my new Doctor's surgery almost feeling like a teenager. Having just received excellent results about my present state of health, I had every reason to radiate joyfulness. It was only four years previous that I had been regularly consuming two bottles of wine, eating fast food like it was going out of fashion and leading a life style either pumped up by adrenalin, or fuelled by stress and frustration. This along with a lapsed fitness regime and months dependant on prescribed Prozac pills I felt sure that I was going to be delivered some bad news about my internal organs and their functionalities.

So what had changed over the past few years for me to breeze through my midlife medical MOT, apart from curtailing the obvious unhealthy habits, which had somehow escalated from 'moderation' to 'excessive' during late 2009 into 2011. I began to consider all the factors which may have possibly been a contribution to the miraculous outcome.

Firstly, I was no longer under continual pressure to achieve targets, however, not just from companies, or managers striving to be ahead of the game, with little concern for the well-being and efforts from their staff, but from my own outrageous, often unachievable objectives too. It is one thing to have high standards, hopes and aspirations, it is another when we try to reach for the stars without the ability to enjoy what is already obtainable. I advocate being busy, I have always thrived better if there is plenty to do, but there has to be measures in place so we can build into our lives what is most important too. I do remember a friend saying to me in the eighties *"Never will you have a weight problem, because you are always on the go!"* I proved her wrong many years later, but I do understand what she meant from her observations, however, although I always tried to make time for family, close ones and myself, generally work related matters and the ongoing quest to improve my status always took precedence.

Stress is the number one trigger for most illness, which according to a number of surveys is triggered by two key factors, these being work and money, both were prevalent to my poor mental health, both of which I have over the past couple of years curtailed allowing me to maintain a much more benevolent and healthier lifestyle. It is not easy to be authentic in a world where becoming second in a race is never quite good enough, but the only steps I will consider to take in my present career, are the ones that feel right in my heart. Being a winner, being the best at what we do isn't such a bad thing in itself, however, whilst we are entrenched in the belief that a pillar of society is merely based on his or her excess wealth, countless properties and endless material possessions, this will continue to breed a selfishness that overshadows compassion and kindness towards others. In reality, all around the world there are many who are suffering, barely able to make ends meet, some living on the streets without homes, children going without meals because of poverty, so how many winners can there be and how many losers have to suffer because of this increasing possession led mentality? What a difference the world would be, if we listened to our inner soul instead of constantly seeking to impress others through possessions, status and wealth.

Secondly, my continual pursuit of materialistic acquisitions was ultimately replaced by my childhood passions, alongside other values and likes which had changed dramatically. I much preferred spending my leisure time walking along a quiet lakeside enveloped in nature, rather than drowning in the hustle and bustle of busy department stores. My desire to be seen in the swankiest wine bars trying to pertain my posture in six inch heels, whilst sipping champagne had more than diminished in favour of a stroll along the beach, feeling the sand between my toes.

Spending time with nature
Sunset walks just by the sea,

*Replaced the endless shopping trips
with loaded bags a guarantee!*

*Walking barefoot in the sand
The grains rest between her toes,
The six-inch heels have disappeared
Along with the fancy clothes!'*

Thirdly, since choosing to become vegetarian in February 2014 the increase in my vitality and spirit was unquestionable. It hadn't been a particularly hard decision to make, because lamb, duck and rabbit were never part of my diet and I had barely eaten red meat for years. The choice to stop eating animals was quite simply due to my concern with the increasing cruelty linked to factory farming. The meat industry seems clouded by the competition within supermarkets, driven by immoral and inhumane practises to sustain gluttony, profit and greed, with little thought for the basic needs of the animals involved. My conscience would no longer allow me to contribute to another living being's unnecessary suffering.

Lastly, the daily meditation had to have played a crucial part in my bountiful wellness. Since May 2012, apart from the odd day here and there, I had been determined to keep up the discipline. The benefits to my mind alone were amazing, but the results from my midlife MOT had to be testament to its powerful effects on the body too. A clear indicator that what we give, we receive, not only to others, but to ourselves too.

It was also in late 2014 when I came to the conclusion that I needed to change my speaker identity from S.M.Toni. The reason was due to the constant barrage of questions in relation to the name and the confusion it seemed to be causing in reference to what my talks were about. At the time of the decision I had been running an animal welfare petition, which wasn't particularly successful, but from the frustration and anguish over a failing campaign that I had called 'A Compassionate Voice' came the new title for my speaker/writing business. This was when everything started to move so much faster. A new website was created that I could maintain myself by adding blogs and videos of my work, a face book page of just over five hundred members, which had been steadily ticking along with little interaction suddenly gained momentum. Now, with over three thousand followers the page continues to grow, with a large number of postings receiving an incredible number of likes and shares, and so many beautiful comments too. 'A Compassionate Voice' a business name that finally made sense to everyone instantly.

I concluded the year by toasting in 2015 with Jools Holland and his Rhythm & Blues Orchestra at the annual BBC New Year's Eve Hootenanny. I danced like I hadn't danced in ages, with having so much to be grateful for and everything to look forward to, I don't think I could have welcomed in the New Year in any better way.

For the first time in my life, it felt as though I was sitting on top of the world, however, the desire for people to look up at me, applaud my position and admire what I had become no longer seemed appropriate, instead I wanted to encourage and inspire many others to join me, in what I had found to be a far better place to dwell.

CHAPTER 13
NATURE HEALS

"We are standing firm
And we will grow and grow
And we cannot pass this by
Until the minority who seem void of a conscience
Join us to end our fight!"

Two occurrences in my life finally brought home to me what was truly important, both being significant in helping me decide the path I would eventually take.

The first incident was almost four years ago, not long after I had moved in with Mum. This was when I first met Sammie, one of three swans who resided on the lake within the country park I frequented. A beautiful young female swan, I didn't think much about our early morning encounters at first, but as time went by she soon became a close companion and the catalyst to many ideas for 'A Compassionate Voice'.

Back at Mum's I started to live a much healthier lifestyle again, so once more I became an early riser, something I had never fully appreciated, or felt I had the time to enjoy before. Peeping through the curtains at a new dawn was so different to where I had been living, because instead of looking out at a tiny garden surrounded by what seemed like a million houses in every direction, I was greeted instead with scenic views of woodland, fields and a huge old oak tree, home to thousands of wildlife.

Mum's bungalow may be small, but it certainly has its good points. The wildlife is in abundance, Tits and wagtails hover around the bird feeders, which I religiously replenish with nuts, whilst at the same time I always scatter some on the pavers underneath for the visiting squirrels, wood pigeons, blue jays, robins, woodpeckers and nut hatches. We have also had the odd visit from a sparrow hawk, though I doubt his interest was in the nuts.

I remember feeling extremely nervous at being alone during my first early morning walk in the country park, but with each visit the fear subsided and I started to embrace every sound, the different colours, seasons, rain, snow, wind and sunshine.

I would trudge through the woods at least four or five times a week in my leopard print wellington boots, wrapped either in warm layers of winter clothing underneath a walking jacket, brown woollen scarf and matching cap, or tracksuit bottoms and tee-shirts in the summer months. Two hours of peace and tranquillity taking with me a bottle of water, mobile phone and feed for the wildlife, just the bare essentials in a tan coloured shoulder bag.

Wondering between the trees, I became mindful of their various sizes and stature, noticed the robins peering at me through the branches, spotted the squirrels as they quickly scurried out of sight amongst the branches. Every morning was a completely different adventure, a totally changing picture of natural beauty. I've witnessed the sky so heavy with snow it seemed to touch a ground already inches deep from what had already fallen, creating a white canvas effect. Autumn colours so breathtakingly unbelievable, with an eclipse of the sun made even more beautiful by the serenity of the lake and surrounding woodland. Being amongst nature is one place I can guarantee anyone can heal, learn to be mindful and live in the present moment. This was when every book I had read suddenly seemed to make sense. My life suddenly felt as though the last piece of a jigsaw had been found, a piece that had been missing for a very long time and one which was extremely important to the completion of the picture.

As time went on it almost appeared as though the wildlife were becoming familiar with my presence, robins would come out to greet me and squirrels didn't automatically go into hiding. I always assumed it was probably the crunching sound of my feet under snow, or leaves that alerted my arrival, but in theory this should have given them the opportunity to make themselves scarce, so is nature's intuition much stronger than ours? Did the robins and squirrels sense kindness and love through my energy and vibration. I was definitely intrigued and started to do some research finding an article by Maryann Mott written not long after the tsunami in 2005. *'Did Animals Sense Tsunami Was Coming?'* It discussed the behaviour of animals and in particular the wild life up to ten days prior to the natural disaster, questioning if it was animal's intuition and in particular, the wild life that saved so many more of them than human beings.

Sammie the swan was also showing these tendencies too, seeming to realise who I was immediately. As I approached the lake with feed she would look me straight in the eyes, chatter to me with her beak and wag her back tail in delight. Eventually she would step out of the water to greet me, stand by my side, even tugging at my coat sleeve a few times with her beak, until I eventually overcame my nervousness and allowed her to eat from the palm of my hand.

Sammie was such a gentle, beautiful bird, who not only helped me with my recovery, but at a crucial point in my life gave me a sharp reminder of how wonderful unconditional love can be for the soul. A period of time when my emotions were playing havoc with my behaviour, I was making rash decisions, finding it hard to forgive injustices, forget grievances and let be.

'Conditional love isn't easy
And it cannot last for long
With demands and expectations
To sing their every song,
Unconditional love is easy
It comes without the strings,
When there isn't any motive
It's amazing what it brings!'

But it wasn't until August 2014 I realised just how important Sammie had become to me. I hadn't been to the country park for over a week because of a holiday, however, on my return I noticed she was in some kind of distress after taking feed from me. Her beak would not close, she seemed to be gagging, almost choking. Extremely concerned for her welfare I walked over to the park ranger's office, but there was no one there, so decided I would call a national animal charity when I got home. Before I left the park I called by the lake to check on Sammie, the gagging seemed to have stopped and after being assured by a member of the fishing club her injury was being taken care of by a vet I went home relatively happy, thinking there was no need for further concern.

Somehow though, I just couldn't get Sammie out of mind, so decided to step up my visits to the lake in order to keep an eye on her. For almost three weeks the beautiful bird suffered unduly. Firstly, because I had put my faith and trust in others after being assured that her welfare was being taken care of, but much worse than this was the ongoing struggle with a national animal charity and some of the fishermen, who used the lake to practise their pastime. Both continually discredited my diagnosis of the bird, trying to sway me into believing she was in perfect health, however, in my mind there wasn't a shadow of doubt Sammie was deteriorating fast.

Eventually after spending almost a full day by the lake taking videos and pictures of the lethargic bird to prove her suffering, only to be rebuked once more, I decided to find help elsewhere. The problem was I had no idea where to go, or who to speak to. I felt completely overwhelmed, powerless and grief stricken, because I knew time was running out for my beautiful feathered friend, yet I couldn't seem to get her the help that she needed and so rightly deserved. At last my determination paid off when a search of the internet pulled up a number of smaller wildlife sanctuaries.

Within hours Sammie was rescued by the Yorkshire Swan Rescue Hospital, but my ignorance had been shameful to these smaller volunteer rescue charities I could have spoken to in regards to the swan's predicament, particularly after being told on her rescue that she probably would not have lasted much more than a couple of days.

I watched the founder of the charity lift her from the water where it soon became apparent the cause of Sammie's ill health. A discarded fishing line was cutting deep into her lower beak and down her neck making it almost impossible for her to digest, so for over three weeks she had been slowly starving to death.

It was touch and go for Sammie, however, the small group of volunteers at the wonderful North Yorkshire sanctuary slowly managed to bring her back to full health.

I drove up to see my lovely feathered friend during her three-month recuperation, but sadly for me she barely recognised who I was. This was the last time I ever saw her because just as I asked she was released on a lake in Yorkshire, where she could live out the rest of her days more safely.

I have so many wonderful photos of Sammie that I hope

one day to transform into a beautiful framed picture collage, which eventually will hang pride of place in my new home.

For the three years she was in my life she taught me so much about myself, ignited my passion to be a voice for the voiceless, which in turn not only helped me to recover, but also overshadowed my own personal issues suddenly making them feel less important. I have always said she helped save my life, but at the same time I am so delighted that I was able to repay her in the same way too.

To all of you Mummies and Daddies
Can you help me? Help set me free?
I was stolen and taken from Mummy
As we swam in our home called the sea.

Saturday January 17th 2015, I joined over a thousand people in London's winter sunshine helping to raise awareness about the truth behind dolphin and whale captivity. The peaceful demonstration encouraged a wide variety of protester's. Young, old, families, children, teenagers and pets, some in fancy dress, all in good spirits making their way to Trafalgar Square with a message to share. Compassionate, caring people ring-fenced under the varying labels that our leaders of society create in order to protect their domains. Movements and groups very often incorrectly branded to mislead and give the impression they are representing a minority's opinion, when in actual fact statistics can clearly show they are speaking on behalf of the majority of the public.

But January 17th was also the first anniversary of the capture of Angel, a rare baby albino dolphin, who along with Sammie the swan captured my heart, becoming the other kingpin of 'A Compassionate Voice.' www.acompassionatevoice.co.uk

I have loved dolphins since being a child and for a number of years swimming with these beautiful creatures had been listed on my Bucket List, nestled in-between witnessing the Northern Lights and travelling on The Orient Express. Sadly, my ignorance failed to question how these dolphins had ended up in captivity until January 2014 when I witnessed the cruel kidnapping of Angel. Swimming innocently by the side of her mother, she was callously ripped from the sea in Taiji Japan for a life of captivity. Just like many more dolphins around the world she was taken from her natural habitat to fuel a trade profiteering from yet another form of animal abuse.

My heart broke into a million pieces as I was shockingly made aware of the extreme pain, anxiety and suffering these endearing, forever smiling sentient beings were expected to endure in order to humour people at dolphin shows. Their natural playfulness exploited to line the pockets of a few. Once again I had been given verification that my voice was needed for the voiceless, so it was a proud moment for me to speak on their behalf in Trafalgar Square, but it was whilst reciting 'Message from an Angel' within the speech I became completely overwhelmed. Looking out across Trafalgar Square, listening to the almost deafening silence that fell upon the crowd as I delivered Angel's message over the microphone, whilst watching many of the onlookers reaching for their hankies, it suddenly became apparent to me that I could possibly help to raise awareness through my written work. I had penned the poem a few days after Angel's capture in the hope it would reach out to Mums and Dads, who were maybe contemplating taking their children to a dolphin show. Surely my creativity could speak out for many other issues and injustices too.

"If someone had told me a few years ago I would be speaking in Trafalgar Square at a peaceful demonstration I

wouldn't have believed them.

I've loved animals since being a child. I'd watch the cowboy films with my Dad and when the fights broke out with the Indians I'd say 'I hope none of the Horses get hurt!'

Thing is for years I've been marching through life trying to be this person I thought I was supposed to be - to be seen as successful.

It wasn't until unexpected events turned my life upside down I realised the world I was living in was a sham and that's when I woke up to who I really was!

What I am trying to say is people and circumstances change and that's what we are here today for, to raise awareness and encourage the change."

The opening of my speech in Trafalgar Square.

From a little girl I have never questioned my love for every living creature I share the planet with, whether it is a tiny spotted ladybird, or the most majestic of elephants. However, like many more I have lived in ignorance for a long time in regards to the immense cruelty bestowed upon other living beings throughout the world. It takes education, research and understanding before embarking on a crusade, but like a dog with a bone I will never be shaken from what I truly believe is my purpose in life. My intentions are set in stone to do whatever I can, wherever I am able to help the vulnerable and the voiceless.

I am ashamed of humanity's lack of respect for other living being's emotions. What I have witnessed through live streams and pictures on social media over the past few years is beyond cruel, and in the twenty first century is simply not justified. Pilot whales held hostage for days without food in shallow waters before meeting a grisly death. Thousands of farm animals transported for days in cramped conditions without access to basic comforts, just to be slaughtered at the end of their harrowing journey. Bears captured and caged for up to fifteen years to produce medicinal bile and beagle puppies raised purely for experimentation - the list is endless. All prisoners, who have been served a death sentence, having done nothing wrong only to be born without a voice.

The treatment of animals is a sickening outrage, during their often ridiculously short lives many are given no basic privileges, they sometimes never see the outdoors, are unable to smell the fresh air, or feel the warmth of the sun on their backs. Ripped from their families and denied even the smallest grain of happiness. Factory farming, dolphinariums, bull fighting, trophy hunting, all animal exploitation driven by a small minority's thirst for greed and power.

There have been numerous occasions over the past thirteen years I have sat with my pet cat Maddie sharing with her my thoughts, discussing ideas and mulling over problems. Good times, bad times, tears of joy and sadness, she has been content to go through most of my ups and downs. Never has she complained, interrupted, or told me to shut up when I have been discussing with her my latest dramas. There may have been an odd occasion when she has walked away in her cat like manner, with her nose and tail directed towards the ceiling, but more often than not her big blue eyes seemed to be fixated on my every word.

Like all animals, she is unable to speak to me and yet Maddie has found many ways to communicate with her human family, so I fail to understand why anyone would wish to underestimate an animal's level of intelligence, or worse, deny they have feelings. I am sure most pet owners will agree, our fur babies become a cherished part of the family, however, even though they do not have a voice, we can usually tell by their behaviour if they are happy, sad, or feeling poorly.

Our adoration of animals is proven on social media too, where their popularity supersedes celebrities, making them the true superstars of the World Wide Web. There is little doubt that the majority of human beings cherish animals and would not wish unnecessary suffering on any species, so why are they dealt such a cruel disservice all across the world? Because far too many decisions are triggered from the mind, from the ego's perspective, rather than from the heart and we need to help to turn this around. Decisions made solely from the mind encourages greed, competition and power, which is why we have animals sadly labelled as commodities, entertainment tools, pests, trophies and targets, rather than the sentient beings they are, who feel fear pain and stress just like we do.

Most pet owners seem to appreciate their dogs and cats have intelligent little minds. I overheard a conversation a few months ago by two elderly people, who were both walking their dogs through the woods. *"He almost talks to me; he understands every word I say,"* one said to the other. *"I know mine's exactly the same, he seems to know when I'm not feeling well too,"* was the response back.

I had already discovered from Sammie and some of the other wildlife inhabitants in the country park that they too have incredible intelligence, but not only this, they are also probably more intuitive than perhaps we are. What about farm animals though, who are so often painted to be stupid with neither intelligence, or emotion.

I made a decision in early 2015 to visit a Farm Animal Sanctuary, because I needed to witness first-hand what I knew to be right in my heart. I had been a vegetarian for just over a year and was already starting to replace a number of dairy products too, including milk and butter. It was so much easier than I had imagined to buy alternative food products from the high street stores which tasted just as yummy and were equally as nutritious.

Many tests seem to have proven that pigs share a similar intelligence to other species credited for their intellect and awareness such as dogs, chimpanzees, elephants, dolphins, but what about sheep, chickens, turkeys and goats? Should intelligence define a species anyway, or how they are forced to live and die, because just like human beings all these creatures mentioned above, like so many more are born with a heart. A beating heart which is the nucleus of life, a beating heart that is regarded as the centre of our emotions, so why not theirs too.

I could not have enjoyed my day anymore at the Farm Animal Rescue Sanctuary in Stratford. The founder Carole Webb, yet another heroine of mine had decided over thirty years ago to sell up and care for abused, neglected and unwanted farm animals, in particular sheep. All are welcome though at the sanctuary, including the old, blind, disabled, boisterous and young. The small team of volunteer's care for over five hundred rescued animals and birds, including a number of pigeons, one nicknamed Costa which Carole jokingly explained *"Because he cost me a lot of money to mend!"*

Being given the opportunity to bottle feed a couple of the sanctuary's latest residents I fulfilled and crossed off one of the items on my bucket list. Blossom and Jack, two six week old lambs rescued and saved from slaughter by one of the charity's supporters. I made a friend for life in George, a six-month old pig who had been delivered by strangers around Christmas time, the previous year. They had found him in the middle of a road presumably having fallen from a livestock transporter heading for the abattoir. He played with me just like a pet dog would do, leaving me slightly worse for wear, completely covered in mud, but deliriously happy. I met so many four legged personalities on Saturday May 24th 2015 at Farm Animal Rescue Sanctuary that it only reaffirmed to me what I already knew to be true. All sentient beings want to be happy, all sentient beings want to feel loved and most importantly all sentient beings want to live.

Respect, kindness and compassion are not just designated values for human beings and it would be extremely selfish to think they are, but somehow in the midst of a consumer driven society we have allowed gluttony, self-indulgence and materialism take precedence, allowing a massive increase in animal exploitation.

"But there are so many injustices to human beings in the world too!" I hear you scream and you are right, but this is my passion, so knitted together with a strong commitment to helping disadvantaged children, whilst also encouraging wellbeing through nature and compassion, my future plans have never been more purposeful.

One of the organisers of the protest I attended was asked the question *"why dolphins? Surely there are much more important issues around the world to protest about?"* Her response was poignant and resonates with me completely. She suggested that whatever their concerns, or whatever felt important to them, change could only be triggered by actively doing something to effect that change.

So, I would like to make a proposal? Whatever eats into your soul, whatever you feel most passionate about, no matter how many people say you are wrong, regardless of how many people sneer, or laugh behind your back, if it feels the right thing to do and it's going to make a positive difference, then do it. Too many people for hundreds of reasons do absolutely nothing, simply because they think as an individual they have little power to make a difference, but if everyone made a few changes, took some positive steps in altering their life styles for the benefit of others and the planet, the impact would be significant. We cannot afford to leave it to everyone else, we must grab what is important to us with both hands and do something today, so we can guarantee our future generations a much better world to live in. Do we really want to go down in the history books as the human race that screwed things up?

'Now it's time to face the facts
We have a world in jeopardy
'The human race they screwed things up'
Is this the message we'd like to see?'

I have sat so many times on my usual park bench by the lake watching the ducks and geese go about their daily business, whilst the swan glides towards me cutting through the mass of water birds like royalty, looking down on them as though they are the reprobates of the lake.

Over the past few years I have been privileged to witness so much. The seven fluffy little ducklings growing up, every visit nervously counting them one by one, grateful none of them had come to any harm until eventually I could barely distinguish them from their Mum. Talented air displays from seagulls playfully swooping down for bread thrown into the air for them by a regular walker. Sharing several minutes with a robin, one quiet still morning in a secluded woody area. Watching him enjoy the seed I had gently placed on the branch that he was perched on, whilst patiently seeming to pose for my new camera as I desperately tried to work out the settings. Chattered with squirrels when they have stopped to give me the once over, before scurrying across my path towards the nearest tree out of sight.

I have enjoyed the autumn winds blowing across the lake's water, creating ripples on the surface as the cool air also gently sweeps across my face. Jumped in muddy puddles, wrote in the snow and screamed *"life is wonderful"* from a deserted hill top looking down on the town where I live. Nature has been profound in my healing, but also a constant reminder to me whenever I walk, sit or meditate surrounded by its beauty that we are never alone.

"We should always stick by what we consider to be morally right, even if sometimes it feels like we are standing alone."

CHAPTER 14
A NEW BREED OF POLITICIAN

'Politicians with false promises
Laws that don't make sense,
So we've come to this conclusion
We're coming down from off the fence,

We'll be the change we want to see
Reflecting grace to change the wrong,
Guiding goodness, steering kindness
To build a world where love is strong.'

Ashamedly, until a couple of years ago I had very little interest in politics. Most election times I have been a voter, but only because I remembered my Dad's harsh tones, mortified by the one time I didn't. *'What's the point'* I sheepishly said to him *'MPs are all the same!'*

The feeling of despair though after hearing the final result from the UK's election during the summer of 2015 was unbelievable for someone, who for many years could not have cared less which party was governing the country. *'Five more damned years'*, I read the headline news across one of the national tabloid papers from a newspaper stand later that day, nodding my head in agreement.

In my eyes, the wrong party had won the Election, but would any other party have made any difference to my town, this country or across the world? I doubt it and yet the countless times the word *'compassion'* was bandied around in the candidate debates, used as a means to win hearts was laughable. *'Compassion'* obviously scripted into manifesto pledges by their media moguls, encouraging voters to place a cross against his, or her name, as each one fought for the keys to 10 Downing Street.

'Compassion' should be a key element in political decision making, however, it will take more than the word being cleverly marketed into the vote pulling speeches of politicians to address all the humanitarian issues in the UK, let alone across the world. This word's flippant use was sickening when we have so many unresolved problems that could have been tackled sympathetically a long time ago, but quite simply just continue to be ignored.

I watched the critical debate intently, prior to the vote for my country to go to war with ISIS (ISIL). I observed a packed house of commons, busier than I had ever seen it before, even though as a nation we have very little to be proud of with so many children living in poverty, families struggling to pay their bills, an NHS crying out for funding, visits to food-banks at a record high, homelessness on the increase and a substantial growth in mental health problems. These are all important matters that have been escalating for a number of years, but somehow have never been shown the level of importance, or support as the recent fixation and urgency I was witnessing to go to war.

I listened to the jeering, the cheering, flamboyant speeches, some riddled with propaganda, others articulated purely to fatten some of the MPs already inflated egos and it confirmed to me just how desperately this world is in need of a new breed of politicians. History repeated itself once more as a yes vote was declared to despatch our bombing planes, despite the growing concern of the public. A conclusion which seemed to be rushed through without time to take a breath, barely allowing anyone even a moment to think things through clearly, a swift knee-jerk reaction that will once again inevitably put more lives in danger.

"Insanity: doing the same thing over and over again and expecting different results." ~ Albert Einstein

I was flabbergasted at how many MPs had turned up to the debate, however, it also allowed me to notice the male dominance within the commons that day too. A definite imbalance of the sexes, which probably gave a clear representation of the majority of government bodies and company board rooms around the world. Although we do have some women in senior decision making positions, I doubt it is nearly enough to have any major impact at all.

I started to consider the shattered state of our beautiful planet derived from countless years of similar ruling. I pondered at how differently Mother earth would look if we had an even balance of female and male energy working together encouraging more love, creativity and inspiration. Surely, this would help to defuse the lethal cocktail of ongoing destruction to the planet.

Consider my proposals for a few moments, if by the side of all the heads of governments around the world, the banks and huge corporate businesses, which tend to be predominantly male dominated, there were also figure heads similar to Mother Theresa, Dame Jane Goodall or Alice Herz Somer, each with an influence in the decision making, I am certain the changes would be profound. These ladies are simply plucked from my own person list of inspirational women past and present, who have helped me to fully understand how life works best.

I have never been a feminist and although I spent most of my twenties braless, this was more of a fashion dilemma, rather than a wish to make a political statement. My only issues at the time was making sure my strapless dresses and off the shoulder summer tops looked elegant, so casting aside my 34DD holding apparatus was merely a safeguard to stop unsightly bra straps interfering with the appearance. I have no wish to discredit the male population either, because there has been and still are members of this sex who fight tooth and nail for peace, equality and compassion, but at the same time, it is also not rocket science to see our planet is in pretty bad shape with famine, disease, war and inequality all still making headline news.

Compassion has to rank high on any agenda, kicking to one side power, wealth and status, which although has been the driving force in our world for endless years has only proved to encourage the wrong type of selfishness.

Selfishness was described in my mind perfectly by the Dalai Lama on 'World Peace Day' September 21st 2015, when I was fortunate enough to see him speak at an event held in the London Lyceum by a national movement 'Action for Happiness.' In my own words I will try to explain his analogies of the two types of selfish that he labelled on the day as 'wise selfish' and 'foolish selfish.'

'Foolish selfish' is all about me, me and me, which has no consideration for others, therefore if combined with greed and power will encourage exploitation, deceit, and corruption. In the worst case scenario this type of insensitive, self-seeking lifestyle can also inflict suffering, harm, or ultimately death to others. There is never any good comes from this type of selfishness and as a motive it will only ever give short term satisfaction.

'Wise selfish' on the other hand is a much more uncomplicated way to live, because although we must learn to love ourselves, we do it so that we have the strength, understanding and empathy to help others. As individuals we are all capable of 'foolish selfish', however, we can also practise 'wise selfish' too. We can help rid the world of 'foolish selfish' by firstly adapting 'wise selfish' as often as we possibly can, but also by kicking out of our lives some of our habits, actions and impulses that encourages the 'foolish selfish' to take a lead role.

I truly believe there is already an outpouring of 'wise selfish' throughout the world. I reckon the intensity in kindness is growing prompted by the increase in awareness of the many injustices and unnecessary sufferings of all living beings. This gives me so much hope for the future, overshadowing any pessimism triggered by some the decisions made by politicians, or world leaders. Are we seeing the shoots of change from the multitudes of people doing wonderful things for numerous causes and issues? Campaigners, volunteers, activists, defenders, do-gooders, philanthropists, good Samaritans, there are so many descriptions given for the real advocates of compassion.

'From Addict to Activist' has been a past headline to describe my transformation from shopping addict to campaigner and although I wouldn't argue with its illustration of my journey so far, in truth there have been many other facets to my renewed lifestyle.

But one of the best ways I feel able to explain my life up to the present date, is by describing it as having lived on either side of a fence. I feel fortunate for being given the opportunity to have experienced both sides, however, my reluctance to cross over onto the other side took thirty years to do. Fear of the unknown, fear of leaving behind the lifestyles we have grown accustomed to, fear of who we will become, even the fear of losing our identity, whatever that maybe, these are just some of the many reasons we dare not venture over to the other side of the fence. Sadly, even though I thought the first side was the right place to be, I was being guided by 'foolish selfish' for most of the time, therefore swamped with delusion, turmoil and disappointment. I can ill afford to say my time on the first side was wasted though, because this is where I have spent the biggest chunk of my existence so far and the wisdom gained from the lessons learned is irreplaceable.

I find it extremely difficult to understand why I hung around on the first side for so long. What was I doing, thinking and waiting for? A Knight in shining armour perhaps, or six winning numbers on the lottery, neither of which would have made me any happier at the time.

But this is why I believe these movements of campaigners, activists, do-gooders, volunteers, etc. are spreading like wildfire, because people like myself are continually waking up and crossing over onto the other side of the fence, after realising life on the first side wasn't all that it was cracked up to be. Some may realise much sooner than others, whilst there will be ones like myself who could take a while longer, however, as the masses grow so will the encouragement until even those sitting on the fence will climb down, unable to bury their heads any longer. This is how we will affect positive changes in the world, when we unite to put things right and influence a new breed of politician.

CHAPTER 15
THERE IS A WAY

*"Just because it's always been that way
Doesn't mean it has to stay that way!"*

In 1999 I stopped my 20 a day smoking habit and the reason for my decision, I'd simply had enough. From the age of fourteen after sharing a few crafty puffs on one of Dad's flipped cigarettes with my brother, the nicotine dependency began to take hold, keeping me hooked for almost twenty-five years. Starting with packets of No 6, moving onto Benson & Hedges, before finally bringing the curtain down on the addiction after a few years inhaling a milder brand, believing this would be more beneficial to my health.

I even spent a short period of time trying to master the art of rolling my own, buying cigarette papers and loose tobacco, but somehow I never quite grasped the technique, always feeling fingers and thumbs. It was when I was on a train journey down to London to see my favourite band Squeeze, I decided to return back to the simpler life again and buy a packet of twenty cigarettes. A young guy had been watching me frantically trying to battle with paper and loose tobacco, hindered by the motion from the locomotive, which was making it even more difficult than normal. Smiling, he asked me if he could help and within a minute he had rolled it, sealed it and handing it me back. A perfectly even looking tobacco joint, a feat I had never once managed to accomplish, however, although a little peeved I thanked him and graciously accepted his offer of a light too.

I had tried a few times to quit, but obviously couldn't

have wanted it badly enough, because the slightest upset would find me reaching for an unopened packet hidden away in a handbag, or rushing to the nearest local shop in desperation. We seem to think that in comforting ourselves with addictive and often destructive habits such as cigarettes, food, drink, drugs, gambling and in my case spending this will help to relieve our burdens, when all these short term pleasures actually do is dull the way we truly feel for a short period of time. They keep our focus preoccupied on the nonsense, rather than finding the root cause of why our emotions are in tatters and although this way appears a lot easier to deal with, sadly problems never go away if they are not faced head on. In fact, the old saying turning molehills into mountains can be used as a reverse meaning idiom in this type of situation, because problems do have a strange way of developing into huge great whopping complications if over a period of time we deliberately choose to ignore them.

In 1999 I was encouraged for a number of reasons to put an end to the nicotine habit. I was fed up with feeling breathless after climbing a few flights of stairs, sick of smelling the lingering stale of tobacco in the car and living room, even sometimes on my clothes, so I decided it was time to screw up the fag packet and quit, which is exactly what I did. It was late one evening and I had been chain smoking during an hour's long telephone conversation with a friend. I put down the receiver, then clenched my fist tightly around the cigarette packet by the side of the phone. I knew the damage would make the last four filter tips unrepairable, but without any remorse I threw the screwed up remnants into the kitchen waste bin. The following morning I did wonder how soon it would be before I purchased another packet, thankfully though, from that day on I never smoked again.

Family and friends were astonished at how easily I had

chucked the £40/£50 a week habit, never needing nicotine patches or gum, which were the two well-advertised stop smoking aids at the time. I didn't find it difficult at all, only ever succumbing a couple of times to a crafty drag on someone's cigarette after a few beers with friends. The funny thing is once I had decided to stop, even during my biggest heartaches, or the most punishing issues I never once considered reaching for a smoke. I obviously cannot deny that I relied on other alternatives to help make situations feel better, but I still maintain my ease in quitting cigarettes is a clear indication if we want a situation, outcome, habits, the way we feel about our past, or ultimately our lives to change badly enough, we have both the inner strength and the will power to do it. We also have the capability to succeed on our own too, without any assistance from quick fix solutions marketed and sold over counters as the easiest way to defeat whatever it may be we are hooked on.

Social beings we are, so a cooperation is needed within humanity for survival and a united front is the only way we will solve the countless troubles we face within families, in our neighbourhoods and around the world, but we shouldn't confuse this with being dependent on others for our own well-being and happiness either. This is down to ourselves, because no matter how perfect the love may feel we receive from someone else, how incredible a relationship is between spouses, partners, families or friends, life can change in an instant, therefore it is essential we have our own built in mechanism to survive both the ups and the downs. In other words, whilst we can seek advice, ask for guidance and read books, all of which does help, the bottom line is we must make our own choices in the end. It is the only way life works, because if we respond to a decision through peer pressure, bullying, or even by a lack of ingenuity brought on by low self-esteem, it is a guarantee the wrong choice will have been made.

I have always hated being backed into a corner and although I handle these situations a lot more differently now, there was a time when my responsive actions would be in mere defiance. Before packing in the habit I remember boycotting restaurants and cafes that didn't allow smoking in their premises, way before the total ban came into place. Anyone's suggestions that I could probably lead a much healthier life style without cigarettes would be instantly dismissed, digging my heels in firmly, even ensuring I smoked double my usual quota on National No Smoking Day.

"I'm glad the governments have got nothing else better to do than waste money on no smoking campaigns, I will pack up when I am good and ready and not until!" I used to say time and time again.

In hindsight the governments were probably absolutely right to get twitchy about the horrendous side effects of a nicotine addiction. People had been allowed to smoke for years without any indication of the horrific damage it could do to their health. In fact, like many other profitable consumer goods, cigarettes and smoking had been encouraged, even perceived to be glamorous in advertising campaigns.

I absolutely hated the idea of being told what to do. I still feel that way to a certain extent and I am in no doubt there are many more who feel exactly the same way as I do too, so I can almost guarantee that the only way to inspire others successfully is through understanding, diplomacy and love. Seeing both sides of an argument is essential for encouraging a profound change, an appreciation of the knock on effects for those concerned is crucial, as is the benefits they will receive from taking on board the suggestions being made to them. Bully boy tactics, bloody mindedness and holier than thou stances will hardly ever be vote pullers, but yet we so often ignorantly go down this route to try and get what we want from partners, friends and even people we barely know.

We also have to be the change we wish to see in the world first, because without doubt it is far better to practise what we preach, however, *educating* seems a much more palatable word to me than *preaching,* particularly if our own journey has not always been whiter than white.

I have helped vulnerable children for years, been a lover of animals all my life, I hate to see any living being come to any unnecessary harm, or treated cruelly, but like everyone else I am human, which definitely spells '*not perfect.*' This book has given a clear indication of the errors within my life and that is why I am reluctant to condemn others. Strength is gained from hardship and pain, but we can also achieve a better understanding of ourselves and others too, which encourages empathy, rather than judgement. We all make mistakes, sometimes grave ones, but it doesn't mean we cannot change, or that we are bad people. It is far too easy to criticize someone without first listening to their story.

> It's time we all loved one another
> No matter what we see,
> Because appearances are deceptive
> I'm sure you will agree,
> We can never know how the next man feels
> But we should always lend a hand,
> And if we share our love, show compassion
> This will help us to understand,

Regrettably at twenty I bought a second hand fur coat, reeked of moth balls and a size 22, making it far too big and much too long for my size 12 figure. It was only in my wardrobe for a short while, because even though I tried to convince myself the animal had probably died years ago, it still didn't feel right. Although I am vegetarian, for years I toyed with the idea before finally deciding to embrace the change and although I was never a huge meat eater, it was still a part of my diet. I have probably bought clothes that children from deprived countries stitched together for nothing more than food as payment, worn cosmetics tested on animals too. What I am trying to say is we are all probably guilty of many pleasures without thinking first about the consequences behind the choices we have made. Not because we consciously think *"sod the vulnerable, sod child labour and sod other living beings"* but due to our minds making decisions unconsciously most of the time.

We also live in a world which has tried to hide the sinister truth behind how others live, the many children affected by war and famine in far off places, countless victims of sexual abuse, what we eat, how our food, clothes and other commodities are being manufactured, the millions of animals exploited, driven to extinction, stolen from their habitats, killed so manufacturers and building companies can take over their homes. A humane population who have been cleverly desensitised into thinking that what is happening in our world today, is the only way. Taking all this into account there is plenty of scope for people to change, but not through condemnation, by encouragement!

Do I really want to believe I live in a society that is increasingly growing into a *'screw you, I'm alright Jack community,'* no I don't, but this is because I happen to have a strong belief that most of humanity doesn't feel this way at all?

I know the type of world I would wish to live in and I am almost certain this has to be the same dream for the vast majority. I'm also under no illusions that it would need an immensely large miracle to overturn centuries old traditions, beliefs and set ideas within a couple of months, or even years, however, as I am sure readers of this book will have already guessed, I do believe in miracles.

Sometimes I feel so overwhelmed, almost suffocated by the constant barrage of grisly pictures I see on social media, but despite this I still believe each one of us can make a difference. No matter how small we may feel our contribution, we can help change the future for our children and our children's children. Through making more mindful and compassionate choices in our lives, either in our habits, behaviour, consumption or actions we have the ability to create a ripple effect, which will not only touch those around us, but will instinctively have an effect on thousands of other living beings too. Never underestimate the power that we all have within us to create a better world because even if we don't manage to see predominant changes in our life time, it shouldn't stop us from wanting to help start the ball rolling.

My faith in humanity does crumble a little though when I hear about movements, charities and organisations, who are all working towards the same positive goal and yet seem reluctant to join forces. Perhaps stifled by in house politics brought about by investors, slight differences in opinion, or even worse clashes of ego and jealousy, which predominantly is the cause of so many breakdowns in communication. To me unity is our only strength and unless the majority cast aside their disputes and pull together around the world, the minority, who seem void of a conscience, the perpetrators of corruption, immorality and barbarous acts will continue to have the upper hand. There is only one quest for everyone and this is for compassion, happiness and peace to exist amongst all living beings throughout the world, so our sole objective must surely be to join hands and help make this happen!

Over the past two and a half years working as a speaker, I have been privileged to talk in front of numerous engaging audiences about what matters to me the most.

Subjects extremely close to my heart, such as mental health recovery, mental health stigma, well-being and animal welfare. At the end of an event in late 2013 a lady came to see me and whispered in my ear *"That was brilliant, because you are real."* This was one of the biggest compliments anyone could have paid me and thankfully since that day the compliment has been said many times. *'Real'* because I had been completely open about my fears. Fears, which most people hope that by sweeping them under the carpet they will either disappear, or be resolved by an external source. Fears that encourage the same mistakes to be repeated over and over again, because they are too scared to roll back the carpet and face them head on.

I will continue to speak out for mental illness issues, the disadvantaged, the voiceless and the environment whilst ever my heart is still beating, but what I have learned enormously over the past few years through realising my own repetitive mistakes is being hateful and judgemental to other people's opinions, life styles, who I may see as the perpetrators of unjust, immoral or inhumane behaviour, even those I feel have a personal vendetta against myself is definitely not the answer.

Being 'real' can be extremely difficult at times, especially with people who I know have wronged me, so I can honestly say with my hand on heart that I don't always get it right. I also catch myself shouting at the flat screen TV sometimes, particularly if I decide to catch up with the news and I grimace in disappointment knowing there is only one person who is getting wound up and it certainly isn't the presenter, or who he or she is interviewing. Anger, vile words and venomous actions seriously destroy our spirit, so we need to conquer our frustrations by taking a few deep breaths in moments of despair. The ongoing practise of meditation and mindfulness raises our consciousness levels so we are no longer ignorant to our build-up of aggression. We are given a window of opportunity to quash our negative emotions before they become too severe.

We can never be at peace with ourselves until we appreciate our connection to everyone and this doesn't just include our family and friends, it also incorporates people we don't know and those we dislike too. It is also well worth bearing in mind at this point how easily time changes our perceptions of someone, maybe we have a present enemy who yesterday we clearly valued as a dear friend, or perhaps there is a once upon a time foe, who has since been transformed into today's hero.

> *"Our world is from perceptions,*
> *We create images of who people are,*
> *So at any given moment*
> *They change from a hero, to a villain and then a star."*

Everyone has to do what they can in their own way, in whichever manner feels comfortable and most importantly when the time seems appropriate. We may never get everything we want from life, we perhaps will not get everyone to see our point of view, but if we can be the change we want to see in the world, if we take positive steps in our lives towards this, then others will be inspired to follow.

We all have unique talents and abilities, but we must always look to our hearts for guidance. No road is easy, however, once we are on the right track then no matter what anyone says, or how difficult things become, we will continue our journey knowing it's the right one.

I have read hundreds of books about the 'Law of Attraction,' but one theory which my past experiences seem to back up immensely is that like attracts like. We pull into our lives how we truly feel about ourselves and this includes people, circumstances and events, so if we wish to make positive improvements externally, we must believe we are capable of making those changes. How many times do we hear stories about the continual knock backs highly talented and recognised artists, musicians and scientists have received time and time again, with claims it can't be done, or this is the way it has always been, only for them to finally come back and prove their doubters wrong. Someone with true grit and determination, who has a strong enough vision will not be put off by sceptics or dismissive people, because they have hope and whilst ever they have hope they will always find a way.

'We know there's a way
And we can start from today,
'Love' can be the change to all of our lives,
We know there's a way
And there's no other way,
We've already proved that this one deprives!'

CHAPTER 16
ALWAYS CHOOSE LOVE

*"Standing on my tip toes
to peer over a wall,
Being only five back then
I wasn't very tall,
The grass looked so much greener
With lots of room to play,
But love surrounds me on this side
So this is where I'll stay."*

There were many times whilst writing this book when it became extremely difficult, because it almost felt as though I was living and breathing my past experiences once more. Regurgitating daunting memories was good for me in lots of ways though too, as in the reconstruction of my past events it helped me to understand even more clearly that we should always choose LOVE over and above anything else.

However, the LOVE I am talking about is not the worshipping kind, or the type where we fall in love with someone one day, only for the next day to fall back out of love with the very same person because of an irritating habit, or much worse we, or they have been caught out in an infidelity. During my school days I do remember jilting someone after our first date, through the type of jumper he wore to meet me. I had idolised him for months, so how fickle or shallow can love be sometimes. Please forgive my shoddy decision making at that time and if we can blame youth, perhaps hinged with a lack of diplomacy too, I would be extremely grateful. This type of love can only be temporary and even if we manage to sustain a wonderful, meaningful heartfelt relationship with one partner, just as my Mum and Dad did, it can still be thwarted with difficulties, days of animosity and the ultimate heartbreak, when one partner passes from this world to the next, leaving the other behind, once again as in the case of my Mum and Dad.

The love I am talking about is what defines who we are and is seen working at its best during acts of kindness towards others. Helping fellow beings, who can probably only ever repay their givers back with gratitude. It is the type of love generated, which isn't automatically looking for repayment, definitely not steered by the trappings of social climbing, or reward, never swayed by mindless distractions, doesn't provoke jealousy, or revenge and is actually the only answer to a happier, peaceful and unified world.

We can learn a lot about ourselves from reflection, but Social Media has taught me so much about myself too, so although I am proud of a number of achievements through such channels as Face Book, I fully understand from my own personal errors there can also be many pitfalls. The successes of my last few charity events have to be credited to the vast networking options made available through social media, whilst it has also been incredibly fulfilling helping to raise the profiles of other people's charity and business pages too. Equipped with the knowledge gained from my past marketing and sales background, I have found it relatively easy to work out how to draw people's attention to whatever I am trying to promote for others, or myself, understanding the right image will always speak volumes, but the words written are also key.

The words we publish can so often let ourselves down though and is the reason why I created a few rules for myself, which I try to adhere to before posting on any social media. I don't always get it right of course, but having been the victim of some unsavoury postings from others and also either through retaliation, or anger the composer of a few unjustified status updates too, I find complying with my three simple rules helps to reduce embarrassment and any unnecessary pain, or hurt.

1) Never post on social media after drinking alcohol.

2) Never publically post anything in anger, or retaliation.

3) Always think first and read through posts to ensure they cannot be misread, or misinterpreted.

'If a knee-jerk reaction
Is the source of your action?
You can bet it isn't from love,

If the ego kicks in
To compete, hurt or win,
Rest assured it isn't from love,

So if you have any doubt,
Here's the thing to check out
To be sure it's coming from love,

If it's joy you are feeling
Not a hurt you're concealing,
You can bet it's coming from love.'

I grimace to myself when I consider some of my status updates during my dark and troublesome days. Did I really believe people were interested that I was going to take an incredibly long soak in a bath surrounded by scented candles? I doubt it, but perhaps it did spark the imagination of a few undesirables lurking in the dark realms of the World Wide Web, who would then respond to what could only have looked like a desperate damsel in distress. I often wondered why I was littered with friend requests from single men, who were using social media as a dating arena, however, documenting my every movement, meal, thought and emotion was forced to generate some curiosity.

We can certainly learn a lot about ourselves through our public postings, because the way we generally see the world, is the way we see ourselves. There is no better reflection of who we are and what we are thinking than when we look at our own social media time lines.

It's so easy to sit behind a keypad too and tell someone exactly how we feel, far easier to key in words triggered by emotions such as frustration, envy, spite and anger facing a pc, or mobile screen than facing the person themselves. We should always take a few minutes to ask ourselves a few questions first though before publishing, because this could alter the way we are feeling about the grievance. We may actually start to see things a little differently, even to the point of considering the other person's view. Besides, would we seriously say all those things to a person if we looked them in the eye, is it absolutely necessary to tell the world about our outrage, or could the problem be discussed privately. Once we have shared a public status, although it is quite easy to delete, no matter how few seconds it is visible, there will always be someone who has captured the words and stored them in their memory bank. This perhaps doesn't seem such a serious problem, but it is, if it changes that person's perception of who we are, because of what they saw.

I also believe social media can show up flaws in businesses and people, replicating some of our society's presence of mind. Some twitter users are perfect examples, account holders who try to accumulate followers by deception. The times I have been invited to follow someone and obliged, only to find I have been unfollowed a few days later. I ask myself what was the purpose of their action, if only to build up their numbers to make their account look much better than it actually is. Isn't this what's wrong with the world today, but on a much grander scale. The theory that if I can't get what I want quickly enough through hard work, honesty and sincerity, then I will get it anyway by cunning and underhandedness.

Since starting my business in September 2013 my social media platform has grown considerably with A Compassionate Voice and I pride myself in the fact that this has all been achieved through sheer hard work, with a small amount of advertising to reach a wider audience.

Life doesn't seem fair sometimes and I do remember even as a child being envious of my cousin when she received one of the first walking, talking dolls for Christmas. I became so upset because I didn't have one, but soon got over it when she allowed me to play with the toy.

I think we have to come to terms with the fact that we cannot always have everything we want in life, no matter how unjust it may feel at the time, but rather than demonise the world because we believe we have been dealt the short straw, we need to try and understand why it wasn't meant to be. There are probably a million and one alternatives that will result in a far better outcome in our life, which will probably serve us better in the long term, so we should consider all the options available that may help to turn our fate around. We have to be prepared to struggle occasionally, we should always achieve our goals through fairness and honesty and to make our lives feel purposeful we must choose love as our guidance.

During the last two years I have spoken to a wide range of audiences, reached out to thousands of people through my written work, but my journey destination is far from over, or complete. It is a wonderful feeling knowing there is a purpose in what I do and the way it overrides all the stuff I once thought of as important is amazing. I have blamed others for my own unhappiness, possibly brought people into my life because of my delusions, who were probably suffering from their own self-deceptions too, but to accuse anyone for my own negative outlook on life was wrong.

Truthfully speaking during 2015 my share of disappointments was equal to my achievements, but whatever the circumstance I am more driven than ever before, always motivated to push even harder. We cannot afford to wallow in self-pity for too long and neither should we bathe in riotous glory for excess periods either, as this merely gets in the way of our progress. We are only ever as good as our last achievement, so we must never allow too much time for defeatism, boasting or procrastination.

A few quotes I have derived from my life experiences to date are…

1. We can't change who we truly are and we shouldn't try to either.

2. The only time we stop loving is when we lose faith in ourselves.

3. We have to face up to our fears. We cannot hide, or run away from them.

4. Strength can be gained from hardship and pain.

There is little I crave for these days, however, I still have many hopes and countless dreams to fulfil, maybe a slightly bigger home for Mum and I, although my preference these days would be a cottage in the country, as opposed to a mansion in the town.

'Her dreams had changed these past few years
They were completely upside down,

Now a cottage in the country
Not a mansion in the town!

Enough income to finally wipe my debt clean would also be incredible, because this will allow me to achieve my ultimate goal, transforming 'A Compassionate Voice' into the charity I have dreamed about over the past twelve months. My ideas list is bursting at the seams, each concept waiting desperately to be incorporated into future exciting projects, however, the charity will be certain of its mission, to unite children with animals and nature. Children are the ambassadors of the future, so for me, it is of paramount importance that we educate them about our connection with all living beings and nature.

I have never been scared to step outside the box, but in October 2016 I have another challenge to conquer. Probably one of the biggest endurance tests I have undertaken yet and it was triggered after seeing the founder of Animals Asia, Jill Robinson speak in Birmingham during her visit to the UK in the Summer of 2015. Inspired by her passion and ethics, which resonated with me on every level, I knew immediately I wanted to help the charity.

There could have been no greater challenge for Jill, when she founded Animals Asia in 1998, five years after an encounter with a caged bear on a farm in southern China, which changed her life forever. She learned that bear bile could be replaced by herbs, so vowed to put an end to bear bile farming. Since then the charity has rescued hundreds of moon bears in China and Vietnam, who have lived in tiny cages, sometimes for over fifteen years for their bile extraction.

So, on October 12th I will be boarding a flight from London to China to embark on a five-day trek walking for up to seven /eight hours a day along some of the remotest parts of the Great Wall of China, hopefully helping to raise funds for this wonderful charity.

It isn't rocket science to realise what little time we really do have on this wonderful planet called earth, and particularly as we grow older time seems to pass by so quickly. The months seem to blend into years, so it certainly makes sense to spend this precious gift of life as wisely as we can. We do need to be extremely wary of expecting too much too soon though, because spending time establishing what will truly make us happy, is a far better option than grasping frantically for solutions. Events, circumstances and people don't always knit together as we expect them to, but as I have learned in more ways than one, patience coupled with tenacity will always produce the right answers.

I hope I am lucky enough to live to a ripe old age, but no matter when it is time for me to leave this world behind, even though I may not have conformed to what society expected of me, neither becoming a wife, or a child bearer, I pray I will have fulfilled enough of my future dreams to recognise that this was the reason for my own incredibly unique journey.

I have sympathy with anyone who is suffering from any mental health disorder, because it is a burdensome task trying to explain to anyone without experience, or knowledge, of how torturous living with the illness can be. For over thirty years the disease held me prisoner, however, it hasn't gone away, because from time to time it still tries to swoop down on me, wanting to catch me unaware at every golden opportunity, but my awakened consciousness through meditation and mindfulness now gives me the upper hand.

It hasn't been easy to tell a story that has travelled across three decades and then just as I turned my first half century culminated into the most life changing experiences, however, I believed the best place to start was from the beginning, which is exactly what I did. Retracing my steps from childhood to where I am now has enabled me to see what was hidden for many years behind my own personal issues, whilst at the same time hopefully it will help many others to overcome their own particular hurdles. My deepest wish is for everyone who reads this book to be inspired enough to take action and realise while ever we have hope and love in our hearts, there will always be a way!

Today, my life feels almost complete and because I never give up, I still wonder if there may be someone waiting on the side-lines for the right moment to enter into my life. A special person I can share my remaining years with, who will love Sharon Bull for the person she has now become, but always was.

'While we have hope, there will always be a way!'

For further information about A Compassionate Voice, future events, or how to book me as a speaker please find my website details below. Please also find listed the charities website addresses that I have discussed within the book.

http://www.acompassionatevoice.co.uk/
https://www.justgiving.com/Sharon-BullACV
https://www.animalsasia.org/uk/
https://dolphinproject.net/
http://farmanimalrescue.org.uk/
http://www.ysrh.org.uk/

CHAPTER 17
A COMPASSIONATE VOICE

ALWAYS CHOOSE LOVE
PAGE 149

THERE IS A WAY
PAGE 150

UNITE TO PUT THINGS RIGHT
PAGE 153

A LAND OF PROMISE
PAGE 155

FOR LOVE
PAGE 158

MESSAGE FROM AN ANGEL
PAGE 160

LIFE IS BEAUTIFUL
PAGE 162

EVERYTHING CHANGES
PAGE 164

THIS CHILD
PAGE 166

WALK HAND IN HAND
PAGE 169

TAKE A TIP FROM NATURE
PAGE 170

PEACE MAKERS
PAGE 173

THERE IS AN ANGEL WATCHING
OVER ME
PAGE 175

STEP OUTSIDE THE BOX
PAGE 177

THINK OF THOSE (IT'S
CHRISTMAS TIME) PAGE 178

ALWAYS CHOOSE LOVE

Standing on my tip toes
to peer over a wall,
Being only five back then
I wasn't very tall,
The grass looked so much greener
With lots of room to play,
But love surrounds me on this side
So this is where I'll stay.
©2014 Sharon Bull

THERE IS A WAY

Our hearts feel like lead,
The papers fill us with dread
It's the thought of the misery and pain,
The increasing conflict,
The hurt that we inflict
Can only be classed as insane!

We fight with each other
We destroy, not discover,
We kill, we maim, we command,
We let others suffer
So we can look tougher,
We pillage, we extinguish, we demand.

And the gasps and the sighs
As we see through our eyes
The devastation we cause to our land,
The majestic we cull
So that pockets are full
From the sale of ivory and fur to look grand.

And why is it we feel
That it's okay to steal

The dolphins that live in our ocean,
For pure entertainment
We allow their containment
With no thought for their hurt or emotion.

We cull and we hunt
With the excuse to confront
Our protection from diseases and threat,
But the only contamination
Is man's ego inflation?
And this will sadly be our biggest regret.

We believe God is our role
With the need to control
Every creature, the land and the sea,
We domineer and we boss
With disregard for the loss,
Yet the right way is to love and let be.

Because we know there's a way
And we can change from today,
We can help to enrich other's lives,
We know there's a way
There is only one way,
We've already proved that this one deprives!
Whilst we live this old way

Limitation will stay
Yet there's more than enough to go round,
If greed continues to breed,
Is seen as a way to succeed
We're as doomed as the earth's sacred ground.

But we know there's a way
And we can start from today,
'Love' can be the change to all of our lives,
We know there's a way
And there's no other way,
We've already proved that this one deprives!

© 2013 Sharon Bull

UNITE TO PUT THINGS RIGHT

From far away we hear their cry
This cry lays heavy in our hearts,
Our conscience pricks
The image sticks
How can we pass this by?

From far and near we feel their fear
This fear lays heavy in our hearts,
There's no greater quest
To be addressed
There is nothing more severe!

And we are standing firm,
We will grow and grow,
Because we can no longer pass this by,
Until the minority, who seem void of a conscience
Understand they can't deny,
Their actions shame,
But we will not blame
We unite to put things right,
Until the minority who seem void of a conscience
Join us to end our fight!

From far and near their ordeal is real
This ordeal has touched our souls,
And it's now hard to hide
Behind greed and pride
It's no longer easy to conceal!

From far away we witness their terror
This terror has touched our souls,
And though hard to bear
Together we swear
We will rid this human error!

And we are standing firm,
We will grow and grow,
Because we can no longer pass this by,
Until the minority, who seem void of a conscience
Understand they can't deny,
Their actions shame,
But we will not blame
We unite to put things right,
Until the minority, who seem void of a conscience
Join us to end our fight!
© 2015 Sharon Bull

A Land of Promise

I stumbled on a land
Where I had never been before,
My mouth it fell wide open
As I looked around in awe.

The trees looked so much greener
The blossom and flowers grew,
And everywhere spelt 'Promise'
Because everyone there knew.

Humankind was smiling
No one looked downbeat,
And everyone was equal
But shared something quite unique.

Money wasn't heard of
Countries were all one,
And there wasn't need for leaders
And starvation had long gone.

A land which had no status
But where each had a role to play,
Where crime was in the dismal past

With no thoughts to disobey.
Where children slept with nature
Could play together without harm,
And every animal had their place
Amidst its beauty and its charm.

I stumbled on this land
And whilst I gazed around to see,
I noticed every happy face
And that included me.

There was no need for fighting
Wars just didn't exist,
And the ancient style of compete to win
Showed no signs of being missed.

Everyone worked together
Joined in life's construction,
Finding ways to heal the earth
Without senseless, mad destruction.

And no one searched for glory
Because no one needed fame,
As everyone was special
Therefore, everyone the same.

So is this the land of promise

Where life begins again,
Where everyone has looked within
And decided now's the time, not when.

Where nations pull together
Where people make a stand,
Where love replaces leadership
Where peace holds out its hand.

© 2014 Sharon Bull

FOR LOVE

For children crying without a Mum who understands,
For every being who suffers pain from human hands,
For all the soldiers armed sent out to kill and maim,
For those tormented, who feel trapped by guilt and shame.

For innocent victims whose lives are cruelly taken,
For poorer countries to be enriched and not forsaken,
For those made hostage in a terrorist's game,
For peaceful solutions that will help replace the blame.

So please - for loving kindness to all children let there be,
And for every animal that is chained to be set free,
For peace to end all wars and those to start
And for loving kindness to find its way inside our heart!

For evil and corruption to be replaced by all that's good,
For mental illness in all its forms to be understood,
For the disabled and disadvantaged to be respected,
For our dying lands and species nurtured and protected.

For loving compassion to overpower what greed commands,
For politicians and world leaders to join hands,
For life's natural beauty to be adored above all things,
And for every being to flourish and find their wings.
So please - for loving kindness to all children let there be,
And for every animal that is chained to be set free,
For peace to end all wars and those to start
And for loving kindness to find its way inside our heart!

© 2014 Sharon Bull

MESSAGE FROM AN ANGEL

To all of you Mummies and Daddies
Can you help me? Help set me free?
I was stolen and taken from Mummy
As we swam in our home called the sea,

My family around me were murdered
My Mummy she died of distress,
And now I am held in a prison
Being trained to do tricks and impress.

I don't understand why you hate me
But your actions imply this is so,
My only wish to be with my loved ones
The ones who will help me to grow.

To all of you Mummies and Daddies
Can you help me? Help set me free?
I was stolen and taken from Mummy
And now I'm held in captivity.
I'm confused as to why I was taken

And why you must torture and maim,
I may be a baby albino
But my family did treat me the same.

I can tell you that dolphins and orcas
Feel torture to help raise your smiles,
Life in your tanks is a struggle
As our home spans hundreds of miles.

So, to all you Mummies and Daddies
This is how you can help set us free,
Tell your children the message from Angel
And let's change this world's destiny.

Because it may seem like we are smiling
But in fact we are incredibly sad,
We are lost without our homes and our families
And the freedom of life we once had.

© 2014 Sharon Bull

LIFE IS BEAUTIFUL

Be always optimistic

See the good in all the bad,

As to be so pessimistic

It can only make you sad,

Never hate the haters

This will only eat your soul,

Lessons are translators

To enrich and make you whole.

Look for all the beauty

Where you can't complain,

A smile that is off duty

Only helps to fuel mundane,

Be gracious and forgiving

Learn by each mistake,

Be thankful you are living

What a difference it will make.

Be always optimistic

See the good in all the bad,

Be creative, be artistic
Be whatever makes you glad,
Bury grievances with laughter
Share loving words instead,
All your dreams go after
Never fear what lies ahead.

© 2012 Sharon Bull

EVERYTHING CHANGES

Everything changes
Unlike a picture in a frame,
It helps if we remember this
Nothing stays the same,
People come, people go
Sunshine can turn to rain,
It helps if we remember this
Nothing stays the same.

Everything changes
Unlike our world within,
It helps if we remember this
So we can take life on the chin,
People come people go
Sunshine can turn to rain
It helps if we remember this
Nothing stays the same.

Everything changes
These are lessons that we learn,

It helps if we remember this
It reduces worry or concern,
People come people go
Sunshine can turn to rain
It helps if we remember this
Nothing stays the same.

©2014 Sharon Bull

THIS CHILD

For a Mother to breathe her last breath, in front of her child,

For the child to witness her slaughter, where they belong in the wild,

For this child to be captured, for this child to be chained

For this child to be bull hooked as a way to be trained

For this child to be whipped, for this child to be stripped

Of dignity, family,

For this child to be shipped

Across waters or skies, for this child to perform

To bully, chastise, for this child to conform.

For this child to live in a cage

For this child to lament

In a home made of concrete,

With no grass, just cement.

For a Mother to be denied of her child at the moment of birth

For the child to be slaughtered, its life without

meaning, or worth

For this child to be brutalised, for this child to be euthanized

For this child to be ripped from the umbilical cord,

For this child to be minced, I am truly convinced

Our humanity has a defect — we are flawed.

For this child to be orphaned, for this child left alone,

For this child to be denied of everything it's known,

For traditions that should have been long left behind

For healing notions and potions - come on are we blind,

Because the truth in well being

It needs none of this,

Its compassion and kindness which will lead us to bliss.

For a child to grow up believing life is all about profit and gain,

For the child to be numbed to other being's feelings or pain,

For this child needs to grow consumed in wonder and awe,

To see nature's beauty

But not through an old image passed down from before,

For this child needs to treasure, needs to cherish and care

For this world to survive this child must be aware,

The capabilities we have to reverse what's been done

To understand our power isn't at the end of a gun,

For this child needs to be mindful, compassionate and kind

To know all lives are precious and that we are all intertwined.

© 2015 Sharon Bull

WALK HAND IN HAND

If I was to walk in your shoes
I perhaps would not get very far,
This journey is only for you
And makes you the person you are.

If I was to tell your tale
I'd simply portray with my views,
This is a story created by you,
My story is the one that I choose.

Yet should we walk hand in hand
In an adventure totally unplanned,
One journey would strengthen as two,
There'd be nothing we couldn't pursue.

And if we swapped shoes on the way
Taking care, we each didn't stray,
Understanding would then commence
As our stories begin to make sense.

© 2013 Sharon Bull

WE SHOULD TAKE A TIP FROM NATURE

The robin never worries when
He might see me again,
He doesn't fret or check the time
Neither does the Tit or Wren.

The squirrels carry on with life
So do the Ducks and Swan,
They love to see me when I'm there
But soon forget me when I'm gone.

They never fear they'll go without
They never cast a doubt,
Their instincts tell them what to do
They know what life's about.

They cross a bridge as each one comes,
Seem grateful for my seed and crumbs
But if I'm not there, they worry not,
They don't twiddle their thumbs

Or lose the plot.

They find their food through natural sources
Use their skills when fear forces,
But once its past they never dwell
They don't settle in a worry hell.

We should take a tip from nature
Time is something they never waste,
They see each moment as a token
Yet never rush, do things in haste.

Take their time to build foundations
With ease will overcome frustrations,
They seem to know just what to do
And give little thought to complications.

They take their life from day to day
Don't harbour grudges, find time to play,
They don't waste their time in fear or dread
With thoughts of what might lie ahead.

Perhaps we all should take these tips
It might help us overcome the blips,

So between the clouds we see the sun
Instead of worrying if the rain has done!

© 2013 Sharon Bull

PEACE MAKERS

We don't want to rule the world
We just want to see a change,
We want decisions with compassion
Not with pound signs at close range.

We are sick and tired of wars
Fighting talk and discrimination,
Across all corners of the world
Less starvation, more salvation.

Politicians with false promises
Laws that don't make sense,
So we've come to this conclusion
We're coming down from off the fence.

We'll be the change we want to see
Reflecting grace to change the wrong,
Guiding goodness, steering kindness
To build a world where love is strong.
We don't want to rule the world

We just want to be peace makers,
We're done with greed and poverty
Through with bullies and the takers.
Let's unite and show our strength
Be the change we want to see,
In solidarity let's show humanity
Let's help to end this misery.

Now it's time to face the facts
We have a world in jeopardy
'The human race they screwed things up'
Is this the message we'd like to see?

Now's the time to turn things round
We need to change this legacy,
We don't want to rule the world
We only want to set it free!

© 2014 Sharon Bull

THERE IS AN ANGEL WATCHING OVER ME

There is an Angel watching over me

Of that I can be sure,

It seems as though she's guiding me

Unlike she has before,

She's pointing out directions

Towards a path I need to tread,

She may have tried many times before, but I obviously misread,

She's smiling as I follow all the instructions she has made,

And sighs with much relief because this time it's not delayed.

There is an Angel watching over me

Of that I can be sure,

She steers me where I need to go

And opens each locked door,

She seems to know the answers to every problem I must face,

I'm hoping she will stick around to help me just in

case,

So if I stumble on my journey

She will be there to dust me down,

If a take a different turning

She will correct without a frown.

There is an Angel watching over me

Of that I can be sure,

It seems as though she's guiding me

Unlike she has before,

I want to say I'm grateful for all that she has done

I believe she helped me see the light

And welcomed in the sun,

She smiles because I follow all the instructions she made plain,

We both sigh with much relief at all the happiness I gain.

©2012: Sharon Bull

STEP OUTSIDE THE BOX

Why is it that we wonder, ponder and peruse?
Instead of getting on with it
Lighting up the fuse,
Triggering the notion
Birthing the idea,
But instead of getting on with it
We deliberate the fear.

Born to be creators, instigators and ignite,
Let's make the world a better place
By broadening our sight,
Look for opportunities
Be stronger than an ox,
Inspire and dare to lead the way
Just step outside the box!

© 2014: Sharon Bull

THINK OF THOSE (IT'S CHRISTMAS TIME)

It's Christmas time
PLEASE think of those,
With little income to dispose
On yuletide goodies, festive treats,
Toys and gifts, or even sweets.

For some families Christmas will intrude
As they can ill afford to buy their food,
Clothe their children, heat their home,
Or for some it's on the streets they'll roam.

It's Christmas time
PLEASE think of those,
Who's loved ones vanish and know ones knows
Without a trace, but just in case,
The posters placed to show their face.

For some families Christmas is a chore
When they have children out at war,
Will prayers be answered, will fighting cease
With siblings back and in one piece,

It's Christmas time
PLEASE think of those
Whom through a loss their life has froze,
Past festive times, memories taunt,
With perfect moments back to haunt.

For some their Christmas feels a sham
With thoughts that most don't give a damn,
Low in spirits and without any cheer
In isolation they hide in fear,

It's Christmas time
PLEASE think of those
When the crackers pull and the vino flows,
As we tuck into our festive meal,
Let's think of others and how they feel.

So this Christmas time let's think of those
And share our love in the hope it grows,
Let's sprinkle joy, deliver peace
And pray for suffering now to cease!

© 2013 Sharon Bull

Printed in Great Britain
by Amazon